IT'S *NOT* ALL IN YOUR HEAD

Chronic pain has been called the silent epidemic. But the pain is not imaginary—it is real. Simple daily tasks become exasperating and agonizing. And the emotional side-effects can be debilitating. But chronic pain can be controlled. This remarkable book outlines a unique, drug-free approach to controlling chronic pain, emphasizing hands-on techniques such as relaxation, exercise, and hypnosis. Dr. David Corey examines the relationship between anxiety and pain, in addition to weighing the pros and cons of a variety of treatments. The result is a comprehensive and straightforward book that may make the difference between living in pain or freeing yourself for life.

DAVID COREY earned his Ph.D. in Behavioral Psychology at York University. He currently heads the Behavioral Health Clinic in Toronto and lectures frequently to both professional and community groups. He has contributed numerous articles to medical and psychological journals. STAN SOLOMON writes on health issues.

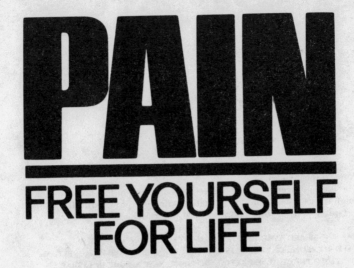

PAIN
FREE YOURSELF FOR LIFE

Dr. David Corey
with Stan Solomon

Foreword by Hamilton Hall, M.D.

Illustrations by Lori McKay

A PLUME BOOK

NEW AMERICAN LIBRARY

A DIVISION OF PENGUIN BOOKS USA INC., NEW YORK

Note to the Reader
The ideas, procedures, and suggestions contained in this book are not
intended as a substitute for consulting with your physician. All matters
regarding your health require medical supervision.

NAL BOOKS ARE AVAILABLE AT QUANTITY DISCOUNTS WHEN
USED TO PROMOTE PRODUCTS OR SERVICES. FOR INFORMATION PLEASE
WRITE TO PREMIUM MARKETING DIVISION, NEW AMERICAN LIBRARY,
1633 BROADWAY, NEW YORK, NEW YORK 10019.

Pain was previously published in Canada
by Macmillan Canada Limited.

 PLUME TRADEMARK REG. U.S. PAT. OFF. AND FOREIGN COUNTRIES
REG. TRADEMARK—MARCA REGISTRADA
HECHO EN BRATTLEBORO, VT., U.S.A.

SIGNET, SIGNET CLASSIC, MENTOR, ONYX, PLUME, MERIDIAN
and NAL BOOKS are published by New American Library,
a division of Penguin Books USA Inc.,
1633 Broadway, New York, New York 10019

LIBRARY OF CONGRESS CATALOGING-IN-PUBLICATION DATA
Corey, David.
    Pain : learning to live without it.

    1. Intractable pain—Treatment.   2. Pain.
I. Solomon, Stan.   II. Title.
RB127.C69   1989   616'.0472   88-32947
ISBN 0-452-26258-5

First Plume Printing, May, 1989

1 2 3 4 5 6 7 8 9

PRINTED IN THE UNITED STATES OF AMERICA

To my wife, Jill, who asked all the right questions

Foreword

For most chronic pain patients, learning to live without pain seems like an impossible task. Because they don't know where to start or how to proceed, most pain sufferers can't solve the problem alone. Dr. David Corey is an expert in helping those victims of chronic pain return to a painfree lifestyle and his programme in Toronto has an enviable record of success. During the many years I have known and worked with David, he has taught me a great deal about the causes, effects and management of disabling pain. Now Dr. Corey has drawn together many of his ideas and techniques and presents them in this book.

His approach emphasizes the difference between hurt and harm, and provides practical ways to keep pain from taking control of your life. New concepts about the nature of pain have led him to new methods of treatment. Two keys are a positive attitude and active patient participation. Pain reduces function. Recovery, therefore, requires physical reconditioning as well as an ability to relax and change your perception of pain. Although every patient needs an individual programme, Dr. Corey has provided here the basic elements and essential strategies to give many pain patients their first insight into their own problems and the ability to initiate a pattern of healthier behaviour.

This is a book based on practical and successful experience. It addresses difficult issues ranging from malingering, lying about the presence of illness or pain for secondary gain, to medication abuse. It destroys the myth of the pain personality, making it clear that any of us in certain circumstances can become victims of the chronic pain syndrome.

Resolving chronic pain is not easy. Acute pain, the natural and even beneficial response to injury, is a part of life. Chronic pain, in contrast, is a damaging behavioural response, a response which is learned over time and bears little or no relationship to the original trauma. It is a behaviour which can only be reversed through knowledge, understanding, and positive action, through recreating patterns of normal activity in a carefully structured fashion. Accepting Dr. Corey's message and putting his ideas to work may make the difference between living in pain or learning to live without it.

Hamilton Hall, M.D.

Contents

List of Diagrams

PART
I

Why We Hurt —
The Human Body
and Pain

CHAPTER 1

Chronic Pain:
The Silent Epidemic

Is constant or recurring pain a part of your life? Or do you know someone who suffers from chronic pain, pain that just won't go away despite the best efforts of his or her doctors? If so, this book will be of great interest to you.

If you've been putting up with pain for many months, you're probably feeling very frustrated and uncertain about the future. Your doctor may have told you that you are healing well but your pain is persisting or worsening. Or you may have a painful disease that cannot be cured. Perhaps the doctor has told you, "You are just going to have to learn to live with it."

If your doctor cannot account for all your pain, he or she might even have hinted that it is all in your head. But you know that you are *not* imagining the pain — it really hurts. It is a frustrating experience indeed. Many patients have told me, "If only I knew and understood why I have this pain, I could learn how to beat it." As I will discuss later, this anxiety only perpetuates the chronic pain, because it causes you to "tense up", and tensed muscles cause more pain.

The strategies discussed in this book can help you with any chronic-pain condition. For example, you may have one of the following problems:

- arthritis (rheumatoid, psoriatic, osteoarthritis)
- post-shingle pain (post-herpetic neuralgia)
- chronic back pain (degenerative disc disease, lumbar strain, mechanical back pain, chronic sciatica, etc.)
- soft-tissue pain (myofascial pain, ligament strains, muscular spasm, etc.)
- generalized body pains (fibrositis syndrome, fibromyositis)
- chronic neck pain (whiplash, cervical strain)
- migraine headaches
- muscle tension headaches
- facial pains (temporomandibular joint pain [TMJ])
- neuralgia pains
- chest wall pain
- abdominal pain
- shoulder-hand syndrome
- knee pain (e.g. chondromalacia patella)

Each of these conditions has one thing in common — pain. And this book is about how you can take control of this pain.

Chronic Pain: An Unacknowledged Malady

"Chronic pain disables more people than cancer or heart disease," according to Dr. J. J. Bonica, who is the father of modern chronic-pain treatment. He was the first to tell doctors that their focus on healing disease was obscuring their ability to alleviate pain symptoms. In Seattle in 1954, he founded the first pain clinic in North America. Since then there has been a proliferation of these clinics around the world. And yet, the magnitude of the chronic-pain problem is still not fully recognized in our society. Why is this?

First of all, chronic pain is not a life-threatening condition like heart disease or cancer or AIDS. With the exception of the occasional drug overdose or drug side effect, no person's life is significantly shortened by this problem.

Secondly, although mankind has always suffered from chronic pain, it has seldom been considered a problem in its own right. Instead pain has been viewed only as a by-product of a disease or other medical condition. Because doctors take this view, patients themselves are in the habit of thinking about their problem in terms of diseases. For example, you hear people say, "I have fibrositis," "He has degenerative disc

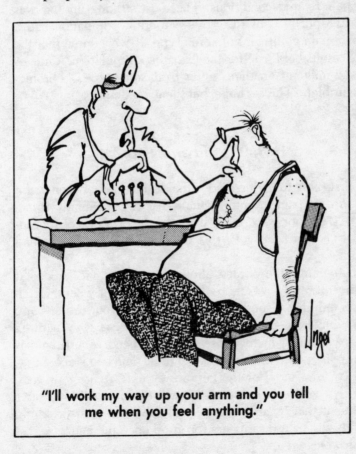

"I'll work my way up your arm and you tell me when you feel anything."

Only you *can feel the pain.*

disease," and "My uncle has rheumatoid arthritis." They don't realize that this way of thinking obscures the common denominator, which is *chronic pain*. Only when experts began studying chronic pain as a field in itself were major strides made in defining, understanding, and treating it.

How many people actually do suffer from chronic pain? In 1985, a survey called the Nuprin Pain Study was conducted in the United States. In this telephone survey, 1,254 adults around the country were asked various questions about pain and pain-related conditions. The most striking finding was that 12.8 per cent of the American adult population had a chronic-pain complaint of some type. If we assume that the same results hold true for the Canadian population, it means that 3.2 million Canadians suffer from some type of chronic-pain problem. This is a huge, but silent, epidemic.

What Is Chronic Pain?

The first thing to understand is the distinction between *acute* and *chronic* pain. "Acute" actually has two meanings. It can mean "sharp" or "severe," or it can be the opposite of "chronic" — i.e. short-term. In this book, I shall use the second meaning.

Acute pain is temporary, although you may not think so at the time; it rarely lasts more than a few days or weeks. Often it lasts only for seconds, as when you stub your toe or bang your funny bone. It is a signal that something is awry, nature's way of telling you to pause and take heed. Acute pain is usually sharper in intensity than chronic pain and is accompanied by an arousal of the nervous system. Acute pain may require a visit to a doctor, who will examine you and offer treatment that, in most cases, will solve the pain problem. Usually the pain disappears for good once the injury or disease has cleared up.

Unfortunately, there are times when that does not happen.

When the medical experts have done their job, but the pain lingers on, what happens then? If the problem persists for more than six months, it is usually classified as *chronic* pain, and it requires a different therapeutic approach.

Let me explain acute and chronic pain by way of analogy. You get into your car and start up the engine. A signal or a computerized voice reminds you to fasten your seat belt. Acute pain is like that reminder — a warning signal. But what if the signal or voice continues long after you have fastened your belt and it cannot be silenced? Chronic pain is like that signal. For some reason the pain-control mechanism remains activated even when the message is no longer useful, and the message itself becomes the major irritant. If you can imagine what it would be like to drive all day with a grating buzzer reminding you to buckle up, you can begin to understand what it is like to suffer from chronic pain.

Some chronic-pain sufferers develop their problems after an accident, usually at work or in a car. Sometimes the injuries that initiate the chronic pain are serious and at other times they are relatively minor, as in the case of a soft-tissue injury. One of the most common problems is chronic low-back pain. After a low-back injury, most victims are better within six months, but there is an unfortunate group of people whose pain continues for many years. For this group of chronic-pain sufferers, it appears that the longer they have the problem, the less likely it is that it will ever go away by itself. Studies have shown that after the problem has persisted for two years, it decreases by itself in only fifteen per cent of the cases. But you can do much better than this by learning pain-control strategies.

What Is Chronic-Pain Syndrome?

Many people function reasonably well with a chronic-pain problem. Others suffer from a more complex and disabling problem known as chronic-pain syndrome. Not all chronic-pain sufferers develop chronic-pain syndrome. How do you know which category you fall into?

I put the following questions to all my patients in our first session and their answers help me determine whether or not they fall into the "chronic pain" category and, if they do, whether or not they can benefit from my mode of therapy.

1. Have you been experiencing pain for six months or longer?
2. Has pain recently spread to new areas?
3. Have you noticed any sleeping disturbances and fatigue?
4. Do you find that strenuous activities, such as cutting the lawn or vacuuming, cause severe increases in your pain?
5. Do even mild activities, such as walking or sitting, cause pain increases after a short period of time?
6. Do you notice that you are gradually doing fewer and fewer things and letting others take over?
7. Have you tried unsuccessfully to return to work?
8. Are you losing interest in sex, perhaps because it increases your pain?
9. Have you been told by specialists that there are no further medical or surgical procedures available for your condition?
10. Has at least one doctor told you, "You are just going to have to learn to live with it"?
11. Are you taking multiple painkillers or tranquilizers, and finding that they are not helping a great deal?
12. Do you find that you are becoming more irritable, are more easily upset, and lash out at others?
13. Do you find yourself often thinking about the accident or disease that is causing your pain and wondering what the future holds for you?

14. Do you sometimes wonder whether others really believe that you have pain?

15. Do you often feel like crying or otherwise feel sad or depressed?

If you answered "yes" to question one and to seven or more other questions, your pain problem falls into a category known as Chronic Pain Syndrome (CPS) and you ought to seek the type of specialized help for this condition that is discussed in this book. Don't despair; there are solutions to your problem.

If you answered "yes" to question one and to between four and seven other questions, your pain problem could develop into CPS in the future. It would be to your advantage to learn the techniques in this book that will help prevent this from occurring.

If you answered "yes" to question one and to fewer than four of the remaining questions, you seem to be managing your pain problem. When we see patients like you, we advise them that they can benefit by learning some special pain-control techniques, but they are already coping reasonably well.

By the way, if you are wondering whether some of the questions are more significant than others, the answer is no. Let me stress that chronic pain is accompanied by many factors which, when working together, produce chronic-pain syndrome. Certain factors that are vitally important to some people, such as work, sex, or recreational activities, are of little significance to others. So my questions are not meant to be weighted in any manner, except that the presence of pain for more than six months does indicate that it has become chronic.

You may also be wondering if all the issues raised in the questions will be treated in this book. These topics are certainly important and will be fully explored in subsequent chapters.

Diseases That Cause Chronic Pain

Before moving on, I want to make clear that if you suffer from a disease or condition like rheumatoid arthritis or sciatica, you should use care when applying the strategies described in this book. You should always discuss with your doctor whether or not these strategies are the treatment of choice for you. It may be unrealistic to think that you can dispense entirely with your medication and other traditional medical treatments and replace them with these techniques. The strategies in this book do not cure disease! Nor do they eliminate the need for good medical care.

However, even in those cases, you can augment your treatment plan with the cognitive-behavioral pain-management principles that are discussed in this book. Just be sure to discuss the plan with your doctor first to be sure that no harm can result.

Learning to Live Without It

What you will read in the following chapters is a different, comprehensive approach to pain control. It will help you to minimize your discomfort and to maximize your quality of life without the need for surgical or drug intervention. For some of you, pain can be eliminated. For the rest of you, your pain can be substantially reduced. Most of you will be able to increase the range of activities you can comfortably perform and almost all of you will feel better emotionally.

If you *carefully* and *systematically* carry out the strategies outlined in this book, you should see significant results in one month. You may have to continue the strategies for several months more for maximum improvement, but keep in mind that your goal here is not just to live with pain. Your goal is to live *without it*!

Results from a clinical study of our program showed that

although only twelve per cent of our patients reported that their pain was *totally* eliminated, over seventy per cent of our patients reported success in significantly reducing their pain and increasing their ability to function normally. The successful patients reported that their pain was reduced by half or more on average.

This book describes the *cognitive-behavioral* approach to chronic-pain management and anyone can learn it. That does not mean it is a quick-fix, magical cure. You will have to put time and effort into the program to achieve the desired results. But if you do so, your rewards will far outweigh your efforts. After all, do you want to spend the rest of your life as a chronic-pain sufferer? I am sure your answer is a resounding NO!

CHAPTER

2

It Hurts, Doc!
Why Can't You Fix It?

Most of us think of pain in terms of injury or disease. This is how modern medicine approaches it. Doctors are taught that all symptoms, including pain, are rooted in disease or injury. This approach is called the *disease model*.

The doctor's goal is to identify the underlying cause of the symptoms and then to "fix" the problem. Medical practitioners are quite good at this when disease or injury is present. In fact many of the major advances in medicine have resulted from this premise. Where would we be today without vaccines or antibiotics? I believe that the very success that the disease model has provided has blinded us from utilizing other approaches in situations where the disease model is *not* effective.

That is why modern medicine is less adept at attacking the dilemma of chronic pain. In some cases of chronic pain, disease or injury is no longer present or cannot be identified by present technology. In these cases, since no disease is identified, there is nothing for the physician to cure. In a second group of cases, the pain symptoms are much worse than can be accounted for by an examination of the patient's physical condition. Therefore treatment of the disease alone will not be sufficient to alleviate the symptoms. In a third group, disease or injury is present but it is incurable. Such is the case with rheumatoid arthritis, where modern medicine can control the symptoms but not cure the condition. As you can see from these examples, the disease model is unsuited to the understanding and treatment of chronic pain.

Of course, when a chronic-pain patient first visits a doctor, the usual procedures must be followed to diagnose a treatable disease or injury. It is only after all the necessary diagnostic procedures and evaluations of the patient's physical condition have been completed that the limitations of the medical approach in a chronic-pain case become apparent. Let's look at an actual case study in detail.

All Too Common

Frank (only his name has been changed) suffered almost constant low-back pain as a result of an accident at work. He was sent to an orthopedic surgeon because his family physician was unable to find the cause of his discomfort. The specialist took a history of his complaints and conducted a physical examination. He then ordered a few diagnostic procedures. Once the results were in, he reassured Frank that his condition was not life-threatening and he discussed with him how it could be handled. He told Frank, "I can't find any cause for your pain, so I'm going to send you to a psychiatrist whom I often use in cases such as yours. I'm afraid you are going to have to learn to live with it."

Where did all this leave Frank? Very upset, to be sure. He felt strongly that his pain was not "all in his head", and he did not want to have to "learn to live with it." To him, this was like being sentenced to a lifetime of untreatable pain.

In similar cases, patients are often told, "Your condition

might be corrected by surgery," or "One alternative is to give you painkillers (or anti-inflammatories) to make you more comfortable." These responses would have been disturbing to Frank as well. He did not want to be told that the only viable option to control his pain was medication. Frank would be quite concerned about the adverse side effects of the continuous use of painkillers and anti-inflammatory drugs — and rightly so! And the option of surgery is not all that appealing to anyone, particularly when the condition is not

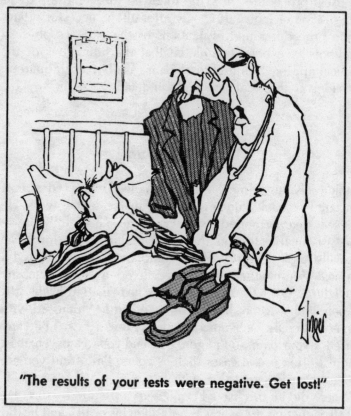

"The results of your tests were negative. Get lost!"

Doctors are stymied when no physiological causes are obvious.

life-threatening and the side effects of surgery are so uncertain and potentially dangerous.

Frank's dilemma is shared by millions of other chronic-pain sufferers, and it is not the doctor's fault! His job is to discover the presence of a treatable disease or injury. And when he doesn't find it, his mandate is really at an end. Very few medical practitioners work in the area of pain management. To the best of my knowledge, there are no courses on chronic-pain management offered in the medical schools.

The typical physician is unfamiliar with cognitive-behavioral pain-control strategies, and is only able to offer such empty phrases as "You'll just have to learn to live with it". The doctors are not heartless; they are stymied. They can only hope that these patients *will* learn how to live with the pain and eventually will battle it down to the point where it no longer controls their lives.

Unfortunately, few chronic-pain sufferers ever figure out how to conquer pain by themselves. The vast majority of them become profoundly discouraged with the final diagnosis of a lifetime of pain or a drugged stupor or both. They have reached the ends of their ropes, and they do not know where to turn next for help. They end up accepting a higher level of pain than is necessary and/or a lower level of functioning than they need to and their personal quality of life gradually deteriorates.

This is what happened to Frank. He saw several doctors about his condition and underwent several treatments, but never found lasting relief or even any answers to his problem. He began to worry that he might have a more dangerous medical condition, one that the doctors were unable to find. He had heard a few stories from friends about people who had suffered similar pains and then later learned that they had tumors in their spines or some other horrible condition. Because of his undiagnosed condition, his pain, and his fear of doing further damage, he gradually became more sedentary and obsessed with his problem. At times he wondered if maybe the pain *was* "all in his head", if perhaps he was somehow doing this to himself as a punishment or because of a flaw in his personality.

At other times he was very angry with the medical profession for failing him in his time of need. Sometimes the anger and irritability produced by his pain exploded into heated arguments with his wife and his family. They came to know when he was in a lot of pain and avoided him at those times. Frank's once happy, supportive family became sullen and increasingly distant from him.

Even his friends stopped coming around. The guys from work called for a few months, but he really had very little to say to them, since he was not part of their group anymore and he was embarrassed about his inability to return to work. Other friends would call him occasionally to go out fishing or attend a sporting event, and he invariably had to turn them down. Even his social life within his own family became strained. Dinners with his wife, going to a movie, or attending a social function became chores instead of pleasurable outings, and he began to find reasons to avoid them whenever possible.

His sleep habits were not the same as before. Instead of falling asleep when he went to bed and waking up rested in the morning, he tossed and turned all night. He began to dread going to bed at night, because he knew he would spend that time worrying about his problems and his physical health. Even though he went to bed earlier than he used to, he still took several hours to fall asleep. Frequently in the night he would be awakened by a stab of pain and sometimes he would get up and wander around the house at 3:00 or 4:00 A.M. while the rest of the family were sleeping. These were the worst times for him, when his mood matched the blackness of the night around him.

It was about this time that Frank was referred to our clinic. When I first saw him, he was wearing a back brace and carrying a cane in his right hand. He leaned heavily on the cane to take pressure off his right leg, so he walked with a slightly stooped-forward movement. He was taking a lot of medication, which made him a little slower in his movements and thinking than he should have been. Emotionally he was vulnerable, and fearful that this visit to another "doctor" would end in as much frustration and disappointment as the previous half dozen had.

By the time I saw him, Frank had become almost completely immobile and sedentary in his daily life. He had not been pain-free since the accident and his pain had spread from the low back to his neck as well as his right leg.

When we assessed Frank's functioning level, we found that even walking with his cane for as little as one minute produced a noticeable increase in pain. Walking without his cane produced the same increase of pain within 37 seconds. Standing without his cane produced pain within 25 seconds and sitting with his brace led to a pain increase within 9 minutes. In order to cope with all the activities that produced pain increases, Frank spent most of the day either sitting or lying in his home. It was obvious that Frank suffered from a severe chronic-pain syndrome.

Happy Endings Do Happen

Discussions were held with Frank and his family to assure them that his condition was not dangerous and that it was treatable. We then designed an individual program for Frank which included all the elements described in this book. It encompassed systematic and carefully managed exercises tailored to Frank's needs by a physiotherapist. He was taught to reorganize his daily activities around the principles of pacing and scheduling (see Chapter 7) which allowed him to control his day-to-day activity rather than allowing the pain to control him. He was taught relaxation techniques, including EMG (electromyographic) biofeedback.

It took many months for Frank to recover from three and a half years of disability and chronic pain, and the effort that he had to put into treatment was quite extensive. Within one month of beginning the program, he noticed that his leg pain began to diminish. (It is often the case that pains more peripheral to the central pain area begin to improve first.) In another month he was able to walk without his cane for three minutes without an increase in pain. At about the same time, he began to attend some part-time courses to help him get back into the routine of leaving his house and interacting with other people again.

In a few more weeks, Frank noted that his leg pains were significantly reduced, and a few weeks after that he was able to discard his cane completely. Once this happened, we began to concentrate on reducing Frank's dependence on his brace. Even short periods without it produced rapid increases in pain, so this was a difficult project for him. And yet only one month later he was able to assume more of the household tasks while his wife was out working, and shortly thereafter he began to accompany his wife to the building where she worked on the cleaning staff. He was able only to assist and not really do much of a physical nature, but it was an important step for him toward vocational rehabilitation.

Six months after starting our program, Frank found a part-time job. By then he rarely wore the brace, and within another month he was able to throw it away. He also started a weight-lifting program under our supervision. Because he had been so inactive for three and a half years, his muscles had atrophied and his level of strength and stamina was much lower than before his accident.

Nine months after beginning our program, he found a full-time job and we were able to phase out our involvement. By this time, Frank's leg and neck pains had disappeared completely. His low-back pain was about half of what it had been before, even though he was doing activities that were many times more vigorous than he could have performed when he started the program. He was sleeping more soundly and feeling more refreshed. He was able to go out with his family and engage in many enjoyable activities, although he still had to be careful to pace himself appropriately. He developed a new circle of friends and started to contact the old ones again. He was particularly pleased with himself when he was able to go on a fishing trip for a weekend. He was now completely off his medication, and was feeling clearheaded and in control now that he was not dependent upon drugs. His confidence began to return and his self-esteem rose.

This is only one true-life example of what can happen with chronic-pain syndrome. You don't have to be as badly off as Frank to benefit from our program. Not all people who suffer from chronic-pain syndrome have low-back pain, nor are all of them so disabled that they cannot work.

Consider Nancy, for instance. She was fifty-five years old, and a full-time homemaker when, several years ago, her doctor diagnosed rheumatoid arthritis. It was particularly bad in her hips and knees. For her, pain was a fact of life. Walking and standing were a constant struggle and there were some days when standing in the kitchen to cook the evening meal was out of the question. Sometimes she had to walk stooped over and it was hard for her to hide her problem from others.

Most of all, the pain affected her enjoyment of life. Instead of being able to participate in activities with her family, such as golfing with her husband, walking down to the beach with her grandchildren, or walking the dog, she was confined to her home and travelling in the car. It wasn't that she couldn't go for a walk in the woods; but the pain that came afterwards made the effort not worthwhile. The anti-inflammatory drugs she took were only part of the solution. What she needed were more skills to enable her to control and cope with the pain.

You will be pleased to know that after three months in our program, although the pain was not absolutely eliminated, Nancy had considerably less pain and was beginning to enjoy life once again. If you also suffer from a form of chronic pain, this book will put you back on the road to enjoying life too.

CHAPTER

3

The Myths About Pain

Before any problem can be solved, its extent must be known and understood. Before an enemy can be defeated, his strengths and weaknesses have to be carefully analyzed so that the proper strategies can be developed. So it is with chronic pain.

"Why," you might ask, "do I have to understand pain in order to control it? After all, I don't have to understand infection before I can take an antibiotic that will cure it."

What You Don't Know about Pain CAN Hurt You!

For one thing, there is no purely "medicinal" cure for chronic pain. That is because pain is the product of the many factors that feed into your *pain system*. The pain system is the sum total of the components of your nervous system (peripheral nerves, spinal cord, and brain) that produce the experience of pain. *Defeating chronic pain means taking an active role in reprogramming your pain system.* In order to do that, you have to examine the components of your pain system, analyze how they all work together, and put the pieces back together in a different way.

Your beliefs about pain are important, because they influence the way you respond emotionally and behaviorally to your pain problem. These responses in turn feed into the pain system. Therefore, the beliefs that you hold about pain can actually increase, or decrease, the amount of pain you feel.

Let's look at some of those beliefs right now. Whenever I ask my patients why people suffer from and complain of pain, I hear the same three basic themes:

1. Most people will tell me right away that pain is related to *physical injury or disease* (including wear-and-tear disorders like osteoarthritis). After all, physical injury is probably the most commonly experienced source of pain, and painful diseases affect millions.

2. I am next most likely to hear that, for some people, pain is purely *psychological* or "all in my head". This viewpoint has been nurtured by the medical profession, particularly when no identifiable medical cause can be found for the discomfort.

3. The third common explanation of pain is *malingering*. People think that others sometimes exaggerate or invent pain symptoms. They feel the sufferer may be motivated by a need for attention or by the anticipation of monetary gain, such as when there is a personal-injury lawsuit or a claim pending against a government or private insurance fund.

Do these ideas sound familiar? You can see that certain beliefs are so ingrained in our upbringing that we accept them as self-evident truths. But look at how inadequate these concepts are. If someone has a pain problem, and is told that he doesn't fall into the first category, he is left with only two other explanations: either he is "crazy" and imagining his pain, or he is malingering or "faking it". Naturally he wants to avoid being classified by others in the latter two categories.

What will he do then? He will look around for a doctor who *will* diagnose a disease and thereby legitimize his pain problem. If this doesn't work, he will become angry and feel misunderstood by a medical system that has failed him. His self-confidence will fade as he begins to doubt his own sanity.

It would be much better if this man understood that his *apparent* options are, in fact, part of the mythology of pain. I am going to tackle some of these myths, because they can have serious repercussions for our ability to deal with the problem sensibly.

The "Hurt Is the Same as Harm" Myth

In the seventeenth century, René Descartes, one of the fathers of modern science, gave scientific weight to the idea that pain was first and foremost an alarm signal indicating harm to a part of the body. The pain signalled an emergency, just as the bell-ringer at the bottom of a medieval church tower rang the bell in the belfry to raise an alarm.

Because of the powerful influence of Descartes's theory, we have come to associate pain most strongly with injury or disease. Since pain frequently accompanies misfortune — as in the case of one being hurt in a car accident or suffering from a particularly painful disease — this theory was readily understood and accepted. We automatically assume that pain indicates bodily harm. The assumption makes sense when the pain is transient or acute. But the same assumption does not apply to chronic pain that continues long after an injury has healed.

What we don't realize is that pain, particularly chronic pain, is not always an alarm signal. The fact that something *hurts* is not necessarily a reliable indicator that a *harm* has been done to the body. Nor is it always accompanied by injury or disease. In other words, "hurt" and "harm" are not synonymous.

A person who believes that her pain is signalling harm will respond with much more anxiety and fear than she would if she understood that it did not signify harm. And anxiety and fear feed into the functioning of the pain system and can actually intensify pain.

Moreover, this person will avoid any activity that increases her pain, because she fears that what hurts is harmful. In her desire to prevent what she sees as damage to herself, she will avoid those very activities related to exercise and work that are instrumental to her recovery from chronic pain.

Doctors can also fall into the "hurt and harm" trap by assuming that a patient does not have "real" pain, or any pain at all, if a disease or injury cannot be found. I have heard a doctor say, "You can't have that much pain. The injury isn't bad enough." This doctor is assuming that he can judge the amount of "hurt" you feel from the amount of "harm" he finds. As you will see in the following chapters, this is a false assumption, which can do more harm than good.

The "Quick Fix" Myth

Medical progress has spoiled us. We expect to take our problem to the doctor and walk out of his or her office with the cure. More often than not, this does happen with an acute problem.

But chronic pain is different. There are, of course, medical situations in which the discomfort is severe and chronic, and drugs and/or surgery are effective: for example, coronary-bypass operations to eliminate anginal pain. But my concern in this book is with chronic-pain problems that are not cured by surgery or drugs.

We advise patients like Frank that there is no foolproof, quick fix for chronic-pain sufferers. But there are other options that work remarkably well in the long run. It is simply not necessary to opt for high-risk surgical procedures or potent drugs with potentially harmful side effects, even if you think you will "go crazy" if your pain doesn't subside. You do have another choice.

Our retraining process is not a quick fix. It can take several months, so you must have patience. However, your patience can be greatly rewarded with remarkable reductions in pain.

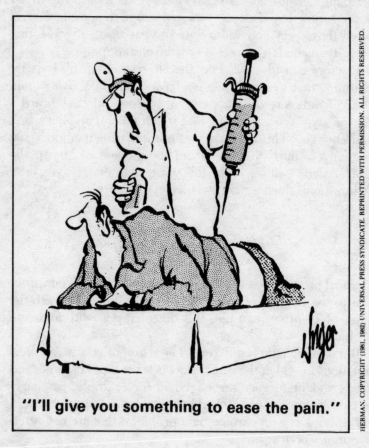

"I'll give you something to ease the pain."

The "Quick Fix" myth.

The "Seeing Is Believing" Myth

When it comes to pain, there are those who believe that "If you can't see it, it isn't there." So, if you complain of pain for which there is no obvious cause — no illness or body damage — these people will quickly question the seriousness of your pain. After all, a person in a cast or a bandage appears to be suffering, unlike someone with an "invisible" problem, such as a headache or a backache.

Medical researchers now know that the cause of a hurt does not have to be seen or directly diagnosed for the pain to be real. A perfect example is *phantom-limb pain*. This is a severe pain that a patient reports in a limb that has been amputated. For many years this pain was thought to be purely imaginary, until more was learned about how the pain system actually functions. Much psychological harm was done to these people by experts who minimized their pain experience and questioned their sense of reality.

You too may find that people don't take your pain seriously because they cannot see evidence of it. The ideas in subsequent chapters may help you to convince them.

The Lingering Myth about Malingerers

Malingering is a variation on the "seeing is believing" myth. There are, of course, people who do fake injuries to collect insurance or compensation monies, or to win a lawsuit. Fakers have been known to quickly don a neck collar to emphasize the seriousness of an injury when an insurance adjuster unexpectedly drops by, but to cast off the device with no ill effects when the coast is clear. However, recent studies indicate that less than ten per cent of all those claiming *chronic* pain are faking their malaise.

It turns out that the majority of "malingerers", as they are known in medical/legal terms, are people who were *recently* injured. It is more rare to find a malingerer who fakes *chronic* pain. Those who stand to gain financially or otherwise from their charade are usually found out before they are labelled chronic-pain sufferers. It is also difficult for them to carry on their theatrics for a long period of time without either wearying of their act or giving it away.

The fact is that there are far fewer malingerers than insurance companies would like us to believe. It appears that over ninety per cent of all chronic-pain sufferers have legitimate pain problems. This is why I start from the assumption that the pain my patients report does exist, even when I cannot see the cause of their discomfort.

Of course, there is a small group of malingerers. There are ways we can distinguish malingerers from those really in distress. You've all heard of insurance companies hiring private investigators to sit in a car opposite a person's house and wait for him or her to start mowing the lawn, fixing the roof, or running for the bus. A more sophisticated method is to collect evidence by watching the patient for inconsistencies in the relationship between pain behavior and reported pain levels. There are ways that malingerers report their pain levels that make me suspicious of the true extent of their complaints. After all, a malingerer doesn't have a problem with pain: he has a problem with the truth.

The "Learn to Live with It" Myth

The belief that people with a chronic-pain condition have no choice but to learn to live with it is perhaps the greatest myth of all. The advice "Learn to live with it" can be the most destructive that a doctor can give a patient. At this point you aren't going to know *how* to go about doing that. These words often produce a sense of helplessness and hopelessness and lead to inaction and invalid-like behavior. What's more, they close you off from the possibility of learning to live *without* it. If a chronic-pain victim is resigned to his fate, no form of therapy is likely to be successful.

How do I know that chronic pain can be alleviated or eliminated, even after medical practitioners have given up? Seventy per cent of our patients attest to the fact that our program works. So when a doctor tells you to "grin and bear it" because he's done all he can do for you, don't despair; it is very likely that you will be in the majority that responds well to *cognitive-behavioral* therapy.

The "Just Deserts" Myth

Many people have been raised with religious or philosophical beliefs that suffering will, in the long run, make them better people. Many believe that God put Job through physical and emotional anguish, and that Job became a better person for it. However, there are not many Jobs in this world, at least not that I know of. For the average chronic-pain sufferer, long-term distress produces disastrous effects on personality, emotional states, and relationships, for a wide variety of reasons.

The Judeo-Christian ethic might lead a chronic-pain sufferer to see his or her pain as a punishment for sin or bad behavior. I have actually had patients say to me, "What did I do to deserve this?" The answer is "Nothing". Seeing their pain as punishment only creates guilt and feelings of inadequacy and serves to worsen the emotional anguish that they feel. These feelings, in turn, can intensify their pain.

Don't Blame It on the Weather!

One of the commonest beliefs about pain is that it gets worse when the weather is lousy. How often have you heard someone say he knows it's going to rain, because he can feel it in his bones? This talent for prediction is most commonly associated with arthritic conditions or low-back pain.

I have observed the pain patterns of my patients over the years to see if there is a connection between the degree of their discomfort and the weather. Why would this be significant? Because you can't control the weather, and if the weather influences your pain, there isn't much you can do about that influence (except move to Arizona). Moreover, if your pain is influenced by factors other than the weather, and you continue to blame the weather for your problem, you may be blind to the real factors at work. Concentrating on the weather prevents patients from looking elsewhere for the real cause of their distress.

In my experience, there is some correlation between pain and the weather only about fifty per cent of the time. The relationship may not always be a direct one, such as dampness affecting the joints. Weather conditions can also influence your moods, and we know that emotions directly affect pain levels. The point is, for the other half of the chronic-pain population, it is important not to blame increased pain on the weather.

Now that you are aware of the major myths surrounding pain, and in particular chronic pain, it is time to critically examine why and how we hurt. So, in the next couple of chapters we will look at the elements that make up our pain system, and how it in turn produces chronic pain. This will set the stage for explaining the cognitive-behavioral method of controlling pain, beginning with Chapter 6.

CHAPTER

4

The Body, the Brain, and the Process of Pain

Trying to explain the reasons why we hurt can be a real headache. Researchers continue to unravel mysteries about the pain process, only to have loose ends multiply and lengthen. Although much progress has been made, particularly with regard to acute pain, the central nervous system continues to guard many secrets. This is especially true for chronic pain, which, as we now know, is quite different from acute pain.

I'm about to take you on a journey through a simplified, but technical, explanation of how pain really works. This will give me a chance to explain some terms and concepts that will appear later in the book. But, most important, until these concepts are second nature to you and part of your belief system, you will not have a framework in which to understand and effectively utilize pain-coping strategies.

Techniques such as relaxation and hypnosis will have only limited effectiveness in controlling pain unless you understand how they actually work to reduce pain. Secondly, you will have difficulty recognizing the influence of outside factors if you do not believe that pain relates to everyday factors in your life. Finally, you will not be as motivated to do exercises or to modify your lifestyle if you think that these things will have little impact on your pain.

Ouch!

The first truly scientific theory about how pain worked was developed by René Descartes. Descartes' theory is nicely illustrated by a drawing he made in 1664 (see Figure 1). His idea was that the heat of the fire produces a response on the

FIGURE 1 *Descartes' Model of Pain*

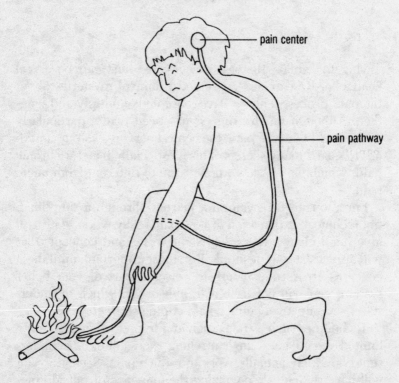

skin of the boy's foot. This action sends a signal up through the body to a "pain center" in the brain. Thus, pain operates as an alarm bell to warn of damage occurring to some part of the body.

This simple theory was widely accepted and has survived the last three hundred years with few modifications. Three important ideas grew out of this theory:

1.   There is one specific pain center, located in a small part of the brain.

2.   There is a single, simple pathway for the pain signal to travel from the site of an injury to the brain.

3.   Pain is a signal for damage only, and therefore there is a one-to-one correlation between the degree of damage and the amount of pain.

Let's examine these three ideas briefly. The first one, that there is only one pain center within the brain, led to some disastrous surgery, in which surgeons cut out specific parts of the brain to try to stop pain. Sometimes they cut out the thalamus; at other times they did lobotomies, severing or cutting out the frontal lobes. This was a dismal failure, as you can imagine. We now know that the pain system is spread *throughout* the brain and the spinal cord, as illustrated in Figure 2. The pain system is interlinked with other systems in the brain that underlie emotions, cognitions, and behavior.

Secondly, as you can see from Figure 2, there are seven different pain pathways that we know about so far, not just one. This drawing shows how complex the pain system is, and we are learning more each year. Even the signals that come from the skin to the spinal cord are transmitted along at least two different sets of nerve fibers. Depending upon which type is more stimulated, it is possible there may be no pain sensation at all in response to a stimulus. For example, we all know the effect of rubbing our elbow after we've banged it against something. The rubbing actually activates the large fibers, which compete with the small fibers signalling the injury, and serves to weaken the eventual pain sensation.

Thirdly, there is no one-to-one relationship between the intensity of a stimulus and the amount of pain felt. Scattered throughout this book are many examples where this supposed correlation breaks down.

Moreover, it is possible to have damage without pain, and pain without damage. In fact, the variability in the relationship between injury and pain is what allows us to intervene to bring pain partially under our control.

It wasn't until 1965 that Descartes's ideas came under question by two pioneers in the field of chronic pain, Ronald Melzack and Patrick Wall. In that year they published a paper called "Pain Mechanisms: A New Theory" in the inter-

FIGURE 2   *Pain Pathways of the Central Nervous System*

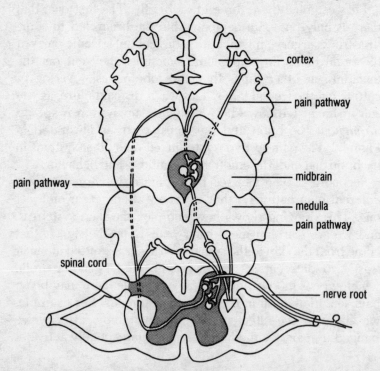

national journal *Science*. In this article they introduced a new model of pain called the "gate control" theory.

The central idea of this theory is that there is a "gating" mechanism in the spinal cord through which harm signals must pass on their way up to the brain. (See Figures 3 and 4.) Depending upon what else is happening in the body or in the brain, these harm signals may or may not get translated into

FIGURE 3   *The Gate-Control Theory of Pain*

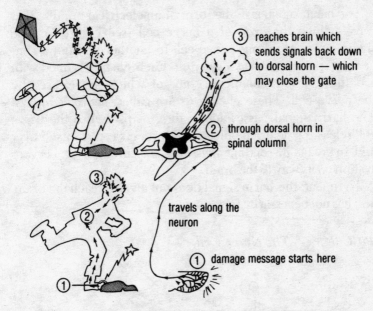

③ reaches brain which sends signals back down to dorsal horn — which may close the gate

② through dorsal horn in spinal column

travels along the neuron

① damage message starts here

FIGURE 4   *Cross-section of Spinal Column and Dorsal Horn which Contains the Gating Mechanism*

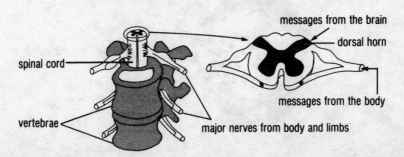

messages from the brain

dorsal horn

spinal cord

messages from the body

vertebrae

major nerves from body and limbs

pain sensations. This theory explains much better the nature of pain, and it helps us to better understand chronic pain.

Thanks to Melzack and Wall, this is what we now know about pain:

1. Descartes was only partly right — a signal *is* sent toward the brain from the site of an injury. But it is not a pain signal, it is a harm signal. And it doesn't always result in a feeling of pain.

The harm signal is in the form of an electrical impulse that travels along the *axon* of a nerve cell (see Figure 5). The signal jumps from one nerve cell to another through a connecting space known as a *synapse*. Each synapse is filled with a bath of various chemicals, some of which are released by the nerve cell. These chemicals are called *neurochemicals*. The harm signal passes across the synapse when the nerve cell releases a neurochemical. This process repeats itself over and over again, sending messages up through the nervous system on its way to the brain.

To repeat, this harm signal does not always reach the brain, and it is not necessarily felt as pain.

FIGURE 5   *The Nerve Cell*

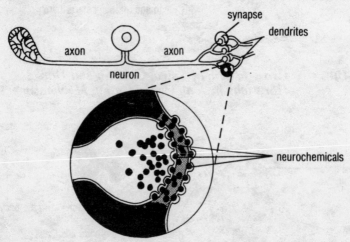

2. Harm signals must compete with other sensory messages. These messages are sent from the injured area as well, and, once they reach the gate, they compete for attention with the harm signals. Since only so much information can pass through the gate at a time, these other messages usually reduce the impact of the harm signals.

These sensory messages are generated by a wide range of stimuli, like heat, cold, or counter-irritation at the site of the injury (for example, rubbing a sore muscle or a banged funny bone). Now you know why you automatically rub an area of your body that feels sore: those competing sensations block out some of the pain sensations at the "gate". Competing sensations also seem to be released by forms of therapy like TENS (Transcutaneous Electrical Nerve Stimulation) or ultrasound applied to the affected area (see Chapter 16).

3. The brain also sends messages *down* toward the gate, and these signals also compete with the harm signals. So, in simplified terms, nerve impulses descending from the brain meet the signals arriving from the extremities of the body at the *dorsal horn* (see Figures 3 and 4), where the gate mechanism exists. Whatever passes upward through the gate will reach the brain.

So far we've examined the main components of the gate-control theory. But this is not the whole story. You may be thinking, "What happens once the harm messages have reached the brain? Do all harm signals become pain? Can the brain produce pain without harm signals, as in phantom-limb pain?" There are still a few more pieces of the puzzle that you need.

The Morphine Within

The discovery of endorphins has helped solve one of the most important mysteries of pain. For centuries, man has known of the powerful painkilling effects of the poppy seed and its derivatives — opium, heroin, and morphine. Medical researchers puzzled over how these chemicals dulled the perception of pain. In the early 1970s, it was discovered that certain nerve cells in the central nervous system were specially adapted to respond to morphine. But why did these nerve cells react to the juice of the poppy? Could it be that there are very similar chemicals in our bodies that just happen to be duplicated by morphine?

The search was on, and within a few years several such chemicals were identified. The first one was called endorphin, or "inner morphine". Related chemicals, called enkephalins and dynorphin, have also been discovered.

These are the body's natural painkillers. They play a crucial role in the pain system, because they are one set of neurochemicals that control the functioning of the nervous system — by being released at the synapses of nerve cells that are part of the pain system. Therefore, the availability of endorphins can play a major role in the production and control of pain.

The release of the endorphins has been shown to have a profound painkilling effect. And, even more important, you can do things to release these chemicals, like exercise and relaxation . . . but more about this later.

The Reign of Pain Falls Mainly in the Brain

The title for this section was coined by a colleague of mine, Dr. Dennis Turk, who is a leading expert in pain research. He believes that the brain holds most of the keys to unlocking the mysteries of chronic pain.

The gate-control theory is not enough to explain the whole pain system. The key to the production of pain is in the brain itself. The brain is "Control Central", where the final decision is made. Sometimes I ask my patients, "If you cut your finger, where is the pain?" They look at me as though I were from Mars, and they reply, "It's in my finger, of course." Unfortunately, even though this seems to be the most obvious answer, it is wrong. *The pain is in the brain!*

I know that we perceive the pain to be in the finger, but this happens to be one of the strange ways that our bodies work. For example, when you see something, doesn't it seem that you are seeing it with your eye? But of course that's only the beginning. The back of your eyeball, the retina, translates the light into nerve signals, which then travel to various places in your brain. The final act of "seeing" occurs within a part of the brain known as the visual cortex. There is a similar process for all of your senses.

Perhaps the best way to understand this part of the pain process is to look at the phenomenon of phantom-limb pain. This occurs in about sixty per cent of people who have had a limb amputated. Many months after the amputation has healed, these people begin to suffer from excruciating cramping pain in the missing foot or hand. How is it possible to experience pain in a part of your body that you don't even have? It's no wonder that for years they were thought to be imagining it.

But recently, with our new understanding of the pain system and the brain, it has become accepted that the brain is producing these pain messages itself. The absence of normal sensory signals from the missing limb seems to permit the brain to produce its own signals. Sometimes it produces a mental picture of the limb as though it were still there (and so the person feels it is there); at other times it produces severe pain.

Another dramatic example of the overall control of the brain comes from surgical procedures that have been used in attempts to control chronic pain. Many persons suffering from chronic sciatica, for example, have chosen to have the nerve fibers that enter to the spinal cord severed. The surgeons believed that this would stop the pain because the signals could no longer reach the brain. Often there was temporary pain relief, but in a few months the pain returned. Sometimes the person was worse off because of side effects of the surgery, including numbness and loss of feeling, and sometimes the pain was worse, too. The surgeons responded to these failures by making even more drastic cuts higher up the spinal cord, but the failure rate remained high.

Even some quadriplegics (who have no sensory input below the neck) experience pain in their lower limbs. Since cutting the nerves here could do no more damage, some surgeons have experimented by removing entire sections of the spinal cord. Certainly, if the pain messages were coming from the body, this should have stopped the pain. But, by now, it should not surprise you that the surgery had no effect. The pain was still felt.

"If pain is in the brain," you may ask, "why don't I get a terrible headache when I stub my toe? Why do I feel the pain in my toe?"

When the brain receives harm signals and translates them into pain sensations, they are then pinpointed on the brain's own map of the body. The message the brain applies to the map-site of the injury produces sensations that we feel as pain back where the injury occurred. The brain does not send pain signals directly to the affected area. I know it *feels* as though the pain is "out there", in your toe. But, in a sense, the brain is playing a trick on you. That is just the way the system has developed and it works reasonably well — except when the pain messages no longer serve a function.

Although there are no pain signals going down from the brain to the toe, the brain does send *motor* messages to the injured site, which act, for example, to tighten up muscles to protect the area. These motor impulses are designed to make you protect an injured area so that the healing process may begin.

This brief discussion of the neurology and physiology that underlie the production of pain is not meant to tell you the whole story, just the highlights to give you the background you need. There are books listed in the glossary that will give you more information on this fascinating topic.

How Chronic Pain Develops in the Absence of Disease

Occasionally, after an illness or injury, the healing process may be complete but the hurt remains. For example, if there is a *soft-tissue injury* (an injury to the ligaments, tendons, or muscles), the tissue usually heals itself within six weeks to three months. But, for approximately twenty-five per cent of those people with soft-tissue injuries, the pain persists beyond this time. After a full year pain will still persist in many of these injured people, and several will have developed chronic-pain syndrome.

This development of chronic pain is very disturbing for patient and doctor alike. No one knows for sure why chronic pain happens, but I believe that there are several possibilities:

1. Sometimes a *vulnerability* remains in the area of the body that has been traumatized, or harmed. The results of physical trauma contribute to this vulnerability. This includes scarring as a result of the healing process, joint stiffness, shortening of muscles, and muscle spasms and weakening.

Scarring and shortening happen most of the time, but some people suffer worse effects than others. Moreover, some people at this point may have an area that is vulnerable to other factors. This means that stress factors the body usually dismisses as insignificant become important players in producing pain. This stress produces muscular tightening and irritation of local nerve fibers, and these messages are then fed into the pain system. Therefore, the vulnerability and the stress, working in combination, can feed a chronic-pain problem in cases where one factor alone would not be sufficient.

2. A second explanation is that of *learned pain*, which is sometimes called memorized pain. An easy way for me to describe this phenomenon is to remind you of those old eight-track tapes (the ones that became obsolete when audio-cassettes and compact discs came on the scene). These tapes

were endless loops that just went round and round, without requiring rewinding.

Now, picture an endless loop going round and round in your brain. But, instead of playing music to your ears, it is continuously producing pain sensation , even though it is no longer receiving harm messages. The original pain-producing barrages have been pre-recorded on this loop, and the brain continues to play them back as pain sensations.

You can learn to override that endless message by programming a replacement. You can also prevent it from happening in the first place, if you understand how it gets started.

One mechanism for learned pain is that of *conditioned response*, which has been studied for many years. For example, suppose a puff of air is blown into a person's eye; it causes him to blink. The procedure is repeated a few times, always with the same result. Then a light is shone into the eye at the same time as the air is blown, and this procedure is repeated a given number of times. On each occasion the person blinks. Finally, the light is shone into the person's eye, but without the puff of air. Still the person blinks, because the brain now makes an association between the light and blinking. Blinking has become a "conditioned response".

Let's now apply this model to chronic pain. Certain people who have strong emotional responses to pain are more prone to developing conditioned pain.

For example, when a person is injured, the trauma produces pain, which is normal under the circumstances. However, during the recovery period, that person continues to experience bouts of pain and emotional upset while she is performing certain everyday activities. Eventually the injury heals, but the pain continues, because the pain system has learned to associate pain with these activities. Through no fault of her own, the person has developed a chronic-pain problem.

Another form of learned pain is *operant pain* which is associated with a reward of some kind. The initial behavior may be spontaneous, but the pain sufferer is rewarded in some way, so the brain remembers the incident and plays it back whenever conditions are right. The rewards therefore serve to initiate and reinforce a learned-pain condition. Two examples will illustrate this.

Ted has chronic back-pain. One Sunday morning he wakes up to find his driveway blocked by a foot of snow. At the very thought of shovelling the snow, he feels his back pain intensify (conditioned pain). He tells his wife about it.

"Don't worry," she says, "Johnny [their son] will clear the driveway. You don't want to hurt your back again."

Ted spends a relaxing morning in bed reading the newspaper and drinking his coffee. He is at peace with the world, but he has established a precedent. His pain behavior has been powerfully reinforced by his family's support, and so has his pain system. He may have his reward, but it is a Pyrrhic victory, because he has developed the beginnings of an operant-pain condition that will be difficult to break.

Another operant-pain scenario is not uncommon. A couple is in a state of marital strife, and the wife, Anna, is a chronic-pain sufferer. The only time the couple do not quarrel is when she complains of intolerable pain. When that happens, her husband becomes sympathetic and solicitous, and the bickering ceases. Anna learns to equate pain with domestic bliss, thereby reinforcing her pain condition.

Let me make it clear that Ted and Anna are not malingerers. They are not consciously exaggerating their pain in order to manipulate their families, even though it may seem that they are. In each case, the pain system in the brain is producing pain because it has learned to do so. The pain that they are experiencing is real and debilitating.

3. The third possibility is that chronic pain may result from neurochemical changes within the central nervous system. While these changes are still poorly understood, the next chapter will help to shed light on the apparent linkage between pain-triggers and the neurochemical functioning of the pain system.

CHAPTER

5

Triggering Chronic Pain

Now that we have looked at some of the erroneous ideas that people hold about pain (Chapter 3), and have summarized some of the more recent discoveries about pain (Chapter 4), you are ready to learn some new and constructive ways to think about pain.

Now is the time to examine what you really believe about your problem. Do you still harbor strong doubts that your doctor is missing something? Do you think, perhaps, that if only a chiropractor or a physiotherapist could place a hand on the "painful spot", the pain would go away? Do you have a hard time understanding that a strong pain in your back can be influenced by stress and anxiety? Do you feel as if your pain is "in the bones" and therefore must be physical and not "psychological" in nature?

If one of the above statements describes your state of mind, you must deal with it now. If it's a second medical opinion you want, go and get one. Perhaps you should find someone who's already defeated a chronic-pain problem and talk with him or her. Or look through one of the books in the appendix that will further explain what I've already told you about the nature of pain.

Let us summarize the things you need to know and believe before you can successfully tackle your pain:

Pain-Triggers

A person with a pain problem must be willing to look at all aspects of his life, emotional state, and personality in order to take control of the pain. This is because factors such as physical activity, pain behaviors, attitudes, emotions, sleep, and stress all play crucial roles in triggering and maintaining a chronic-pain problem. They affect the functioning of the central nervous system and, since pain is in the brain, they can directly modify the final product of your pain system, i.e. your pain.

I call these factors *pain-triggers*, because each of them can trigger the pain system into action. Each pain-trigger can also maintain a pain state, once it has been started, and result in a chronic-pain condition that would otherwise end much sooner. Finally, if one trigger is not enough to fire the system by itself, it can maintain the system in a state of readiness to be triggered by other factors.

This model is illustrated in Figure 6. Note that disease and injury are only two of the many factors that can trigger the pain system. The other triggers are not typically associated with pain, but are just as important, especially in a chronic-pain syndrome.

Everyday experience provides ample evidence of the role that these triggers play in producing pain. For example, almost everyone has experienced the effect stress and anxiety can have in producing a tension headache. In the same way, most of us have experienced how anxiety and anticipation can heighten the pain from even a simple needle jab when we are in the dentist's chair.

Stories about war experiences can also provide dramatic examples. Dr. Henry Beecher was a surgeon in the Second

World War who wrote a book describing his observations on battlefield wounds and pain.

He tells the story about a young American soldier who was part of the invading force at Guadalcanal. It was his first taste of action and he was naturally concerned about his chances of survival. He was very afraid of dying. A few moments after hitting the beach, he felt a sudden sensation of searing pain in his right hip, and of blood pouring down his leg. He collapsed, believing that he had been seriously wounded.

The medics arrived and rushed him to relative safety. But when they examined him, they discovered that only the canteen on his hip had been hit. The fluid he had felt running down his leg was only water. Once he understood this, the searing pain in his leg immediately disappeared. The soldier was quickly returned to the front.

Moments later a mortar bomb landed nearby and he felt a stinging pain in his forehead. When he touched the spot, he discovered blood on his finger. Once more he fell, this time believing he had suffered a serious head wound.

Again the medics arrived and examined him. He had in-

FIGURE 6   *Pain Triggers*

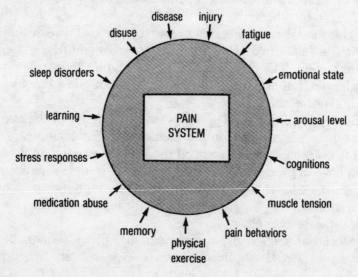

deed been hit by a fragment, but had suffered only a slight scratch on the forehead, which was easily covered by a Band-Aid. For the third time the soldier was sent into the fray.

A few minutes later, another mortar bomb exploded near him and knocked him to the ground. He felt no pain at all, and thought he was fine until he started to get up. Then he realized that his left leg had been blown off.

The point of this story is that this soldier experienced three "injuries", each more serious than the last, but the amount of pain he felt receded as the severity increased. Indeed, he felt nothing when his leg was blown off (though later, of course, it hurt a lot), but experienced excruciating pain at the time of the "non-injury" when his canteen was hit. The factors that triggered his pain had just as much to do with his anticipation and fear as they had with his actual wounds. Just imagine the effect these triggers can have on a chronic-pain problem as they accumulate over time.

There are many stories about how athletes have excelled in the heat of a game unaware of the fact that they have suffered serious injuries while playing. It was only after the game that they began to experience the pain normally associated with such injuries. The reason is not that these athletes are conditioned to "grin and bear it"; they usually report afterwards that they were totally, or almost totally, unaware of the extent of their injuries at the time they occurred. This illustrates the positive side of the equation; the pain-triggers can *reduce* or *eliminate* pain as well.

The Neurochemical Link

There is a physiological reason behind all this, and it is found in the interaction of the chemicals in the brain. These neurochemicals perform an important function in managing the pain system.

When I started graduate school in the early 1970s, there

were only three chemicals known to stimulate nerves at the synapse. Since then, our knowledge of neurotransmitters and other neurochemicals that modulate the action of the nervous system has mushroomed. At current count, over three hundred neurochemicals are known and more are being discovered every year.

As a result of these discoveries, it has become increasingly clear that the brain is not just a giant electrical switchboard or computer; it is also a gland. That is, it produces chemicals that act throughout the body and it also responds to chemicals that are produced in the body. Interested readers are directed to Dr. Richard Bergland's book entitled *The Fabric of Mind* for more information on this subject. For our purposes in understanding pain, it is sufficient to concentrate on only a few of these neurochemicals.

Figure 7 shows a list of neurochemicals (left-hand column) that are known to act within the pain system. Each one has a different role to play. I have already mentioned the role of the endorphins in Chapter 4. Another important chemical is seritonin, which is affected by anti-depressant medication. As we shall discuss in a later chapter, this same medication can reduce chronic pain.

Current research has confirmed the crucial role that these neurochemicals play in the pain system. It is likely that chronic-pain syndrome is associated with complex modifications in the amounts and balances of these neurochemicals.

FIGURE 7   *Neurochemicals and their Relation to Pain Factors*

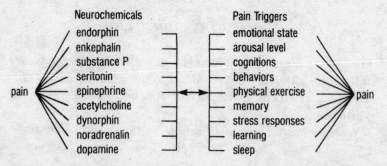

Figure 7 also lists (in the right-hand column), many of the body's functions which are known to be served by these same substances (listed in the left-hand column). For example, dopamine is important to sleep, while stress responses are associated with noradrenaline. Many items listed on the right are associated with more than one of the listed neurochemicals, and vice versa.

It is also important to note that the relationship between the factors and the neurochemicals is a two-way street. That is, changes in the substances produce changes in a person's emotional or physical state. Likewise, systematic changes in one's emotional state modify the balance of the neurochemicals. That important principle explains the control that we can have over the functioning of our own nervous systems, and thus over our pain.

By now you should have noticed that the factors in the right-hand column are some of the same ones that I identified as pain-triggers in Figure 6 of this chapter. This is not a coincidence. In my model the pain-triggers influence chronic pain through these neurochemical imbalances. Therefore, to control our pain we have to control the triggers, and we must do it in a systematic, methodical way.

Pain Is Pain Is Pain

One of the most difficult concepts that my patients have to absorb is that the pain produced by emotions and stress is just as real as that produced by an injury. "Are you trying to tell me that my pain is just psychological?" they might ask when I point out the importance of the pain-triggers. They feel that pain produced this way just isn't as "real" as that produced by physical causes. Perhaps they got that idea from their doctor or it was part of their upbringing, but it is a widespread belief in our society.

At one time, when a doctor wanted to test whether a patient's pain was psychosomatic or "not real", the patient was given a *placebo*. Placebos are fake treatments — for example, medications that are sometimes given to patients who believe they are being treated with real, active drugs. The most common example is that of a "sugar pill" given instead of painkilling medication. The assumption is that those who report getting better after taking a placebo have psychological problems, not real pain.

The placebo response occurs in about one-third of the population. These people are known as "placebo responders". It was once thought that the pain these people were complaining of was imagined, not real, and that's why it went away once the placebo was administered.

However, in 1977 some important research showed that the improvement caused by the placebo was in fact mediated by the release of endorphins, which are powerful, painkilling chemicals. The placebo responders got better not just because they *thought* they were getting real pills, but because of the neurochemical changes induced by the belief. The belief in the effectiveness of the treatment combined with the actual consumption of the placebo induced the brain to release the endorphins. Moreover, the stronger the belief in the effectiveness of the treatment, the stronger the painkilling effect.

This is why, if you believe that the strategies described in the rest of this book are your best choice and that you are capable of carrying them out, you have an excellent chance of learning to live *without* your pain. If you attempt them only half-heartedly, you will have little chance of succeeding. Understanding is the seed of belief, and your belief in your own ability to control pain is fundamental to your success.

All the major pieces of the puzzle are now in place, and we have everything that we need in order to learn the strategies of cognitive-behavioral pain management. The pain system, which is made up of the gate mechanism, the brain, and our neurochemicals, can be modified by the pain sufferer himself. All it takes is hard work — practise and skill and motivation.

PART

II

Toward a Solution
— Strategies for
Overcoming Pain

CHAPTER

6

Introduction to Cognitive-Behavioral Therapy

~~~~~~~~~

In the rest of this book, you will learn how to utilize specific strategies to tackle chronic pain. All these strategies are based on an understanding of the information and principles set out in the first five chapters.

Take another look at Figure 6 in Chapter Five. All the pain-triggers shown there can be approached in specific ways. It is important to recognize *all* of your pain-triggers, because if you deal only with one or two, and there are others that are feeding into your pain system, you will have only limited impact on your chronic-pain problem. For example, I have seen many patients who have had only relaxation training for their pain. They derived only limited benefit because they failed to deal with their pain behaviors, sleep disorder, and physical activity. The point is to leave no stone unturned in dealing with your pain problem.

I will deal with the pain-triggers in the following order:

Identifying Your Pain-Triggers

I've just finished telling you that the first step in treatment is to recognize all your pain-triggers. You will have to initiate this "recognition" process yourself, because it involves determining what factors increase or decrease your pain levels. In order to do this, you will have to measure your pain levels at various times during the day. Only *you* can measure the amount of pain you feel, but we supply the "yardstick" called a *pain scale*.

The pain scale that I prefer rates discomfort levels on a scale ranging from 0 to 10. On this scale, zero means total absence of pain, and ten means the worst pain you have ever experienced, or could ever imagine experiencing. Some people have described having a car door slammed on a finger, labor pain, or a kidney-stone episode as being the worst pain possible. These forms of pain then have become their personal 10s.

FIGURE 8   *Pain Scale*

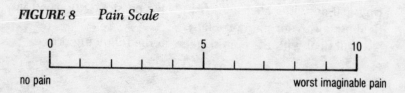

With this scale, it does not matter that one person rates degrees of pain differently than another person would. What matters is that you use the same number to describe the same degree of discomfort on day one as you do on day two. In other words, your rating of various pain levels has to stay the same from day to day.

When using this or any other scale to measure pain, it is important to understand the difference between *pain tolerance* and *pain threshold* levels. We may all experience continuous pain at some time, but can remain fairly oblivious to it, because we are actively engaged in our work or play. We do not notice the discomfort unless we stop to think about it. In this case, the sensation remains below the pain threshold. When this pain increases to the point that it begins to intrude into our conscious awareness, it is at our *pain threshold* level.

When the pain is severe enough to significantly interfere with our activities, we have reached our *pain tolerance* level. At this point we are very conscious of the discomfort we feel, and we are forced to take action to alleviate the distress, such as resting or taking some sort of medication. Between threshold and tolerance, we are aware of the pain, but it does not interfere with our activities.

Patients who are able to identify these two levels are better able to communicate their pain problems to whomever is trying to help them, and to make better use of the pain-rating scale. Also, they are able to describe their distress without having to use negative terms such as excruciating, stabbing, or burning, which only result in negative imaging that perpetuates the pain problem.

Self-Monitoring

Self-monitoring is an objective way of rating your pain at various times of the day, to help you identify pain-triggers and patterns. Let me explain it this way. Before a mechanic

FIGURE 9   Self-Monitoring Form (Blank)

Place: (categories)
H – home
W – work
R – restaurant
Rec – recreation (party, etc.)

Mood: (categories)
A – anxious
B – bored
C – tired
D – depressed

E – angry
H – happy
R – relaxed
O – other (please specify)

Date:

Time	Place	Activity	Mood					Meds
								1
								2
								3
								4
								5
								6
								7
								8
								9
								10

11	12	13		14	15	16	17	18	19	20	21		

Comments:

can begin to repair an automotive problem, he has to understand and diagnose it. He will ask you to tell him where the noise is, when it occurs, and what it sounds like. He has to know all this before he can fix the problem. The same is true of a pain problem, particularly one that is chronic.

When my patients start treatment, I have them systematically record their activities, emotional states, pain levels, and medication intake at various times during the day. The chart below shows how we ask our patients to monitor themselves each day.

Self-monitoring entries are made hourly, from an hour after you get up in the morning until you retire at night. Entries should be made faithfully for two weeks. Every entry should include the time, place, activity, your mood, and medication taken. For ease of use, you can use the following codes, rather than writing out all the details every time.

It is obvious, of course, that you may feel bored, tired, and depressed at the same time. All those feelings, then, have to be entered in the same space. Pain levels are measured on the 0 to 10 scale described above. There is space at the bottom of the page for you to fill in comments about events that happened that day that might help you understand your moods or pain levels.

I suggest that you take a photocopy of the self-monitoring chart on page 54-5 and start to fill it out yourself for the next two weeks. Remember to do it on a regular basis; hourly is best. At the end of each week, you should go back over the charts and comments to identify the factors that triggered your pain.

You might be thinking, "But I've been trying so hard for the last while to ignore my pain. Now you're asking me to pay attention to it. Isn't this going to increase the amount of pain I feel?"

It is true that, at first, patients pay a lot more attention to their discomfort, because they have to fill in their observations every hour. They may initially want to forget the whole exercise, because it is a constant reminder of their discomfort. But think of it this way. First of all, if you've been trying so hard to ignore your pain and it's still there, blocking it out is evidently not a very successful strategy. Secondly, your assignment is like that of the mechanic — you have to analyze the nature of the problem in order to find the solutions.

Once you realize the long-term advantages of understanding the nature of the beast, the very short-term discomfort becomes quite acceptable. Think of it as a little short-term pain for long-term gain.

Analyzing the Self-monitoring Data

The sample chart on the next page has been filled in to indicate the responses of one of my patients. You will notice that the pain levels are quite high in the morning, but drop off quickly after a couple of hours. As you can see, at 3 P.M., the activity of mowing the lawn resulted in increased back pain, while at 7, writing a letter exacerbated her neck discomfort. At 8 P.M. the patient had an argument with her daughter. This stressful event led to a sudden flare-up of both neck and back pain, and the patient became angry. Anger produced more stress, which resulted in even more pain.

During the day, our patient took medication at prescribed times, but there was little relationship between the time the medicine was taken and when the pain flared up or subsided.

By closely examining this day in the life of our patient, we can learn many things. First, certain physical activities aggravate her condition. Secondly, emotional stress can trigger pain. Thirdly, medication and the absence of pain do not always seem to go hand in hand. Much more can be learned from an analysis of self-monitoring charts, particularly when they are compiled for several weeks, when certain trends become more obvious.

FIGURE 10   Self-Monitoring Form (Example)

Place: (categories)
H - home
W - work
R - restaurant
Rec - recreation (party, etc.)

Mood: (categories)
A - anxious
B - bored
C - tired
D - depressed

E - angry
H - happy
R - relaxed
O - other (please specify)

Date: June 8/87

Time	Place	Activity	Mood	Neck Pain	Back Pain		Meds	
9:00	Home	shower	C	9	8			1
10:00	"	breakfast	BC	8	7			2
11:00	"	exercise	R	6	6		2T	3
12:00	Mall	walk/shop	A	7	8			4
1:00	Restaurant	sit	C	6	6			5
2:00	home	lay down	CR	5	5			6
3:00	home	mow lawn	B	7	8		2T	7
4:00	home	lay down	AC	6	7			8
5:00	home	lay down	C	6	6			9
6:00	home	made dinner	CR	6	7		1T	10

Time		Activity				11	12	13	14	15	16	17	18	19	20	21
7:00	home	TV/talk	R	6	6											
8:00	home	talk z daughter	E	8	7											
9:00	home	sit	EA	8	8			2T								
10:30	home	in bed	DC	7	7											
11:00	home	trying to sleep	DC	6	8					1H						
3:00	home	awake thinking about argument	EAC	8	7											

Comments:

T = Tylenol, H = Halcion

I had an argument this evening with my daughter. She said I am having a difficult time since she moved in.

Making Self-monitoring Work for You

After you have completed a week of self-monitoring, you should take a fresh look at the data you have collected. But examine the information as if you were analyzing another person's problem. This detached approach will allow you to be much more objective about your analysis.

Your evaluation will help you discover relationships between activities, moods, and pain that you may not have seen before. You may even uncover other factors you never thought responsible for your distress. Or you may realize that you have been blaming the wrong things for your problems. For example, many people believe that the weather is responsible for much of their discomfort, or for their lack of pain. This may frequently be the case, but, as we have seen, all too often the relationship is a very weak one.

A few years ago a woman who suffered from *psoriatic arthritis* was referred to me. During her first visit, she told me that her worst days occurred when the weather was inclement. Her observation seemed perfectly reasonable, but I asked her to monitor her pain anyway. I also told her to record the weather in the booklet during this time.

She returned to my office two weeks later greatly excited by her findings. The book showed quite clearly that, although she had bad days when the weather was poor and good days when the weather was beautiful, the reverse was also true. What was obvious to this patient, however, was that her bouts of pain always followed arguments with her daughter. The woman had come to realize that she had blamed the weather too much for her woes. Moreover, she knew that while she could not change the climate where she lived, she could do much to alleviate the tension between her daughter and herself. She realized that she was paying too high a price by having her daughter live with her, and she asked her daughter to move out. Their relationship, and her pain, both improved thereafter.

My patient had gained an important insight that comes

from analyzing a pain problem in this fashion. People often see their pain problems on a macro-scale — i.e. as one big picture. The problems seem so overwhelming that they appear to be out of control and beyond remedy. But, if the picture can be broken down into small cameos, it can be made more manageable. This is the "Pac Man theory" of problem-solving — the idea is not to tackle a gargantuan, impossible task, but to break it down into bite-sized chunks, which can then be dealt with separately. Eventually each piece of the puzzle will fall into place and together they will lead to an overall solution of the major problem.

When you analyze the various small "bites" of information in your self-monitoring, you will see the pieces of your pain puzzle more clearly. You are now ready to learn how to best attack your chronic-pain problem.

CHAPTER

7

Physical Activity and Chronic Pain

~~~~~~~~~~

During the initial interview with one of my chronic-pain patients, I asked him what he had been doing for the last few weeks.

"I've been in bed for six weeks," the man answered. "I get up only to go to the bathroom, or to make a meal. This is the first time I've been out of the house since I saw my doctor six weeks ago."

"Why is that?" I asked.

"Well, my doctor told me not to do anything that hurts," the man replied, "and *everything hurts*."

Why Exercise?

The normal response to pain is to stop the activity that causes the pain. This is usually a good idea when pain is acute, because it prevents us from damaging ourselves further. After all, acute pain is nature's way of telling us to slow down and pay attention. It allows our natural healing processes to take over.

But a person suffering from chronic pain is in a very different situation. Rest may cause the pain to abate temporarily but not for long. Moreover, rest has its own penalty, because over the long run you can develop joint stiffness, muscle-shortening and tightening, and weakness. Once this happens, eventual recovery becomes more difficult, because, when the area is finally exercised, pain will result from the stiff and shortened areas. Then it's likely you will return to a sedentary state to avoid more pain, and a vicious cycle will develop.

This is one reason why it is crucial for chronic-pain sufferers to gradually and systematically increase their activity to near-normal levels. As we shall see below, exercising can be highly beneficial if done properly.

The Cart Before the Horse

Most people are used to taking steps toward recovery in a particular order. For example, after surgery, they wait for the symptoms to subside, the scar to heal, the inflammation to die down and their strength to return. Then and only then do they return to all the activities they would normally do, such as exercise, housework, or going back to work.

Understandably, then, people who experience chronic pain believe that they have to rest until their pain subsides before they can try to live normally again. It is not unusual for a chronic-pain sufferer to adopt a sedentary lifestyle in the mistaken belief that immobility will ensure a pain-free state. Some people can be immobilized for a long period of time, and then suddenly jump up and begin exercising in the mistaken belief that they are well again. It is difficult for them to understand that chronic pain is fundamentally different from other kinds of disorders — it does not automatically run its course and then go away for good.

As we noted earlier, a chronic-pain sufferer has an endless-loop problem. His pain behavior and emotional responses feed into the pain cycle. And the pain in turn dictates those pain behaviors and emotional responses. He must break apart this cycle in order to stop the chronic pain. He cannot wait for the pain to go away *before* taking further steps. That is putting the cart before the horse! What he must do is first become reasonably active in order to bring the pain under control.

Easier said than done, you say. True enough. One of our biggest tasks in helping a new patient is to convince her that she needs to undertake physical activities, even though she is in pain and even though the increased physical activity causes more discomfort. These activities, which are not strenuous, may heighten a patient's pain in the short run, but they improve her condition in the long term. Since we are trying to reduce her pain by helping her reprogram her pain system, we must show her convincingly that the link between pain and activity can be broken. That's what this chapter is about.

I want to remind you again that this principle does not necessarily apply to patients suffering from disease processes such as rheumatoid arthritis, in which increased activity *may* lead to more long-term pain and harm. Nor am I referring to acute-pain situations. I am discussing chronic pain only, where the hurt/harm distinction has been clarified by a physician and it is agreed that physical activity will not cause harm.

I differentiate between three basic kinds of activity or exercise:

1. The first type is called *anxiolytic* exercise which is intended to reduce anxiety and tension.
2. Secondly, there is everyday activity, such as household chores, shopping, etc.
3. The third type of exercise involves strengthening, flexibility, and stretching. This is the kind of exercise that you might do in a fitness club or learn from a physiotherapist.

Each of these types is equally important in the reduction of chronic pain. The strategies and principles discussed in the rest of this chapter apply to each of these equally.

Anxiolytic Exercise

Anxiolytic exercises include aerobic exercises — such as swimming, running/jogging, brisk walking, cycling, and other strenuous sports. However, there are other anxiolytic forms of exercise, such as yoga and t'ai chi, which are quite relaxing, though they are not necessarily aerobic.

As I have already mentioned, anxiety can lead to pain when it causes muscular tightening and spasms. One of the best ways of combatting this muscular tension problem is through anxiolytic exercise, which relaxes the body and reduces pain through two mechanisms.

First, it has been conclusively shown that moderately used muscles are less likely than little-used muscles to tighten up. Secondly, there is evidence that sustained physical activity promotes the release of *endorphins*, one of the morphine-like substances that we have in our bodies. This is often evident in long-distance running, where endorphin release is referred to as a "runner's high". This is the stage in any aerobic exercise in which exhaustion and pain subside, and are replaced by a period of euphoria. Is it any wonder that runners become addicted to their sport?

For these reasons, you can use anxiolytic exercise as a pain-management strategy. Long walks, swimming, and similar activities can have a pain-reducing effect and therefore constitute a first, important way of controlling pain. If these exercises are organized and carried out properly, they can help reprogram the brain's pain system.

Daily Activity

Most people who suffer from chronic pain find their activities controlled, wholly or partially, by their pain. They decide whether or not to go to a movie based on how they feel at that particular time. They may put off doing chores around the house. Or refuse an opportunity to play golf with a friend because they "don't feel up to it". They may feel so poorly that they are unable to work, or, if they do, the rest of their lives is undermined by the resulting pain.

Having your life controlled by pain is a frustrating experience. Suppose your back has been particularly bad lately. As a result, you have been watching the household jobs build up over the last few days, waiting for the chance to get at them. Finally, the day comes when you feel better, so you resolve to make a clean sweep of the place.

You spend the rest of the day tackling each job energetically, feeling satisfied that you are finally taking charge. By 4 P.M., you start to notice some strong twinges in your back, and by that evening you are in trouble and rummaging in the medicine cabinet for something strong. After a night of poor sleep you spend the next day back in bed wondering if the satisfaction of the previous day was really worth it and angry that even one day of normal activity is more than you can cope with.

Perhaps you are a businessman who has become increasingly frustrated by your inability to tackle a backlog of work that has accumulated during your bout of pain. You decide to plunge into the workpile wholeheartedly in order to catch up. Like the homemaker in the previous example, you push yourself physically until the job is done, and you end up paying for it, or even end up worse off than when you began. Perhaps you even begin to question your ability to fulfil your work commitments over the long run.

Both these victims have had their activity controlled by pain. They have learned that a particular activity leads to more pain, so they will anticipate this outcome each time they engage in it. This means that their central nervous systems become conditioned by this pain/activity association. Learned pain will therefore become an ingrained part of the pain system.

How can someone begin to undo this damaging pain/activity association? There are three key behavioral techniques that reprogram the pain system and will help you to resume your normal activities: *baselines*, *shaping*, and *pacing*.

The Tortoise Approach: Baselines and Shaping

Suppose Mr. Johnson, a chronic-pain sufferer, is told by his doctor, "Go out and be active." He decides to take a walk to a local park. The problem is that the park is a long walk from his house. By the time he makes it back home, he has reached a very high pain level. So what happens? He's hesitant to try it again because he wants to avoid the high levels of pain. He eventually gives up this walk altogether and begins to settle into an even more sedentary lifestyle.

What this person needs is to learn to *pace* his activities so that he can perform them independent of pain. In order to do this, he will utilize the principles of *baselines* and *shaping*. I will explain all these terms, using the example of Mr. Johnson.

First, Mr. Johnson must establish a baseline for his walk. A baseline is a quantitative measure of the amount of activity that can be performed until there is a noticeable pain increase. In this case, he must begin by noting the time when he sets out on his walk. He should then walk at a normal, comfortable pace until he first becomes aware of an increase in pain (I recommend using a one-level increase on your pain scale as a guide — see Chapter 6). At this point, he should again note the time, to determine how long he has walked up until the pain increase occurs. The total time elapsed becomes his baseline.

In the example we are considering, Mr. Johnson's baseline

was measured in *time* (as opposed to distance). Therefore, the length of his next walk should also be based on time. For example, suppose that at the outset he could walk for ten minutes before experiencing a one-level increase in pain. To be on the safe side, he should reduce his next walk *by half*, to five minutes. He knows almost certainly that he will be able to walk for five minutes without an increase in pain. *For the first time, he will enjoy a planned activity that is not associated with an increase in pain.*

Now for the shaping part. The process of gradually increasing the amount of an activity on the basis of a preplanned schedule is called shaping. I would recommend that he begin by taking several walks a day for five minutes each. This means he walks out of the house for two and a half minutes, and then returns home. After a few days, the walking time can be increased by a minute (in total), or less if desired. During a two- to three-week period of time, the person can gradually build his walks back up to ten minutes — his baseline.

If, during these weeks, he is in more pain one day and feels like staying home, he should *not* break the routine but should continue the scheduled walks. On the other hand, if he feels terrific, as if he could walk for an hour, he should resist the temptation and hold himself to the allotted time. The point is this: if he changes his activities depending on his pain (or lack of it), *the pain is still in control*. If he adheres to his routine, he will eventually find that he can walk for the ten minutes without an increase in pain by the time he reaches his baseline level.

In my experience, most chronic-pain sufferers try to shape an activity too quickly. "After all," they reason, "I used to be able to walk for ten minutes and now I'm only walking for seven. Let's speed up this process." But that thinking can lead to failure. If you shape too quickly, you run the risk of encountering additional pain and falling back into the old routine of having the pain control your behavior. I recommend that you plan on taking two or three weeks to build back up to your baseline. The purpose here is not to finish the activity *per se*, but to reprogram the pain system.

The idea behind the baseline and shaping approach to exercising is that the amount of your activity is now pre-planned. When following this principle, you do not walk until you experience pain severe enough to make you stop or wish you could. Remember, your goal is to disassociate your activity from pain. You want your behavior to become independent of pain so that you no longer anticipate discomfort when exercising. This is a vital step in breaking the link between activity and pain. What we are trying to do is break into the pain system to change or reprogram it.

How far should you shape an activity? The answer is highly dependent upon individual circumstances, but I can provide some general guidelines. Usually you can exceed your original baseline without too much trouble and keep going until you reach a new level of functioning. I have seen people totally overcome their pain using this strategy and go on to jogging and other vigorous activities with minimal pain.

As long as you maintain the shaping principles faithfully and engage in a regular routine, you should be able to greatly extend your ability to perform the activity. Your own activity tolerance depends on many factors, but I find that most people recognize this point readily.

Let us take another example — a person with a back problem who wishes to begin lifting weights again. Using the same principles as with our walker, we start the person off with fairly low weights. When he reaches a weight level that produces a noticeable increase in pain (his baseline), we cut him back to half that amount. Our weight lifter sticks to this low level for a few days, then gradually, but regularly and systematically, increases the amount he is lifting or the number of repetitions he performs.

We call this *working to schedule*. This strategy is markedly different from a commonly advocated exercise principle called *working to tolerance*. When you work to tolerance, you push yourself to your level of conditioning — i.e. when it begins to hurt. This is associated with the phrase "no pain, no gain".

Working to tolerance is not recommended for chronic-pain sufferers. Remember that not only are we dealing with a musculoskeletal conditioning problem; we are treating a dysfunction in the central pain system. We are trying to re-program the brain at the same time.

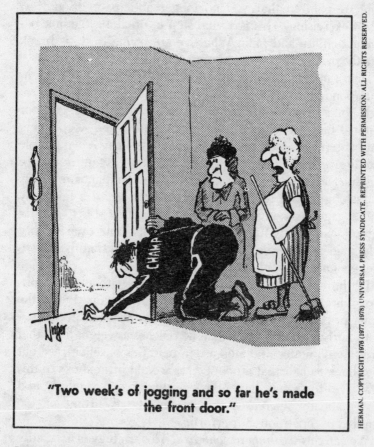

"Two week's of jogging and so far he's made the front door."

Shaping can *be a slow process.*

Remember, the key to success with this approach is to take it *slowly and systematically*. You will recall that in Aesop's fable it was the tortoise and not the hare that won the race.

Pacing: Reining Yourself In

The principles of baselines, shaping, and working to schedule combine to make an effective set of strategies. I like to call this set of strategies *pacing*. The general principles of pacing can be applied to any activity a person may engage in. I have already used the examples of walking and weight lifting. Other examples include sitting, driving a car, doing household chores, and so on. In each case, you must take the baseline, reduce the amount by half, and then shape it slowly. Maintain the schedule faithfully and, when you reach a new plateau, remember to pace yourself according to a schedule that is not dictated by changes in pain.

If you reach such a plateau in driving that you cannot drive for more than one hour before having increased back pain, then remember to stop and take a break before then. If you can't sit at your desk for more than one hour at a time, then be sure to plan your work day so that you can get up and do something else — *before* the pain forces you to. The crucial principle here is not to wait until the pain builds up to the point that it forces you to do something; always plan ahead so that you are preventing the increase and *you* stay in control. Once your pain flares up, it is much harder to bring it under control.

Pacing can be a difficulty strategy for people to learn and apply consistently. It goes against the grain for many who have been taught to "get the job done". For others, who have tried to cope with their pain for many years by trying to ignore it and then push ahead in spite of it, it may seem like they are "giving up". A case in point is an avid golfer whom I treated some years ago. His problem was that eighteen holes of golf produced almost unbearable pain, but he didn't want to give up the game. When I suggested a pacing strategy, he hesitated, saying that playing less than eighteen holes seemed worse than not playing at all. When I pointed out that he might be able to eventually build back up to that point and reduce his pain at the same time, he agreed to give it a try. With the addition of an exercise routine and relaxation strategies, he was able to play a full game again within four months, with virtually no increase in pain.

What about activities whose duration is difficult to control? As you know, there are some things that you pretty well have to complete once you start them, such as taking a shower, making a meal, or working a shift on an assembly line. In such cases, pacing cannot be applied. This is where you will need the relaxation/imagery techniques discussed in later chapters.

So far, I have been talking about pacing according to a predetermined schedule. But there is another type of pacing that you can use. It depends on the existence of a *pre-pain cue*. The pre-pain cue is usually manifested in the form of tightness or mild discomfort in an affected area, and it quite reliably signals an imminent increase of pain. If the pain sufferer is aware of this type of sensation, she can then take it as a cue to cease whatever activity she is engaged in, rather than wait for the pain to become severe before stopping.

The *cue*, rather than the pain itself, thus becomes the signal to stop an activity. By utilizing a pre-pain cue and working to that limit, you will find that you can gradually increase your activity before the onset of the pre-pain cue.

Some people have pre-pain cues but are not aware of them. This is common in the grin-and-bear-it types. They try to tune out all their pain signals, not realizing that some of them are useful. I suggest that you "listen" to your body's signals for a while and see if you don't notice some pre-pain cues. Many people have told me that learning to relax helps them to become more aware of signals from their bodies. Once you can identify the cues which precede the onset of pain increases, these cues can take the place of timing or repetitions on your pacing yardstick.

Pacing as a Way of Life

I suggest that you look at pacing as a whole new way of controlling your life, and your pain. You can adopt a pain-independent lifestyle by scheduling all your daily activities from the time you wake up in the morning until the time you go to bed at night. This scheduling is based on your own plans, not pain. I recommend a three-point program to follow each day.

1. Each evening, prepare a schedule for the following day. It is important for chronic-pain sufferers that there be a consistent pattern to the day. Decide the night before what time you will arise in the morning and what your activities will be. You must be very careful in establishing realistic expectations of yourself. Be sure that you can accomplish all of your goals the next day, even if it turns out to be a "bad" one in terms of pain.

2. The second rule is to schedule rest periods during the day, and to take them at the specified times. Taking a break is not a sign of weakness or of failure; it is a wise move to allow you to gradually build up your conditioning. As you improve, you will be able to reduce the number and duration of your rest periods.

3. Make sure *all* the time periods in the day are filled with activities and rest breaks. You will have to use a daily time sheet marked into segments. When you finish filling it in the night before, every minute of the day should be accounted for. This encourages you to be time-oriented rather than pain-oriented and leaves less time to focus on discomfort. Even rest breaks can become quality periods, because you can spend the time productively in reading or relaxation. The one thing we discourage during these breaks is taking naps,

because sleep during the day can interfere with normal nighttime sleeping patterns.

We always have a few words of caution and encouragement for our patients when they first attempt to set up schedules for themselves. We strongly advise them not to over-schedule their activities, because if they get carried away, they will wind up like our harried business executive who bit off more than he could chew and wound up in worse shape. *You must remember your baselines!*

We also reassure our patients that even though they might not succeed initially in setting up a perfect schedule for themselves, they will eventually get it right. This is important for those of you who will be designing your own routines without expert help. Don't give up if your first attempts at scheduling are not completely successful.

Here is an example of how you might schedule your morning activities when you first begin your recovery program:

7:00 A.M. — get out of bed, shower, etc., and get dressed
7:45 A.M. — make yourself breakfast and read the morning paper
8:30 A.M. — do a few household chores you have on your agenda
9:30 A.M. — take your morning walk
10:00 A.M. — relaxation period begins
10:30 A.M. — call sister about weekend
11:00 A.M. — grocery-shopping
12:00 NOON — lunch

The remainder of the day is similarly broken up into manageable time slots with specific activities and rest periods. As you progress, your rest periods will decrease and your range of activities will broaden.

Scheduling is one of those things that is easier said than done, particularly if you are not a person who can change habits and lifestyle smoothly. But scheduling is extremely important, because it helps to replace bad habits; and this is vital in overcoming chronic-pain syndrome. Once scheduling becomes a habit, you will find it easier to do and the rewards will make it all worthwhile.

De-conditioning

People with chronic pain become out of shape or "de-conditioned" for three basic reasons:
1. Activity is avoided because it is painful (as I have already discussed).
2. Braces and canes are used over the long term.
3. Protective responses develop.

Back braces and neck collars badly weaken muscles in the long run, because the muscles are prevented from doing their job. This is why most doctors advise their patients not to wear back or neck braces for too long. If the muscles in these areas remain unused for a long time, the body comes to depend on the support that these artificial devices provide. Undoing this problem makes recovery all the more difficult.

A similar problem involves the use of a cane or crutches, which are intended to take weight off a painful limb. After prolonged use of these supports, however, the patient will notice that the muscles on one side of the body are weakened, resulting in an imbalance. Also, there is tremendous stress on the upper part of the body, which often becomes contorted or stooped, because of the mechanics involved in walking with these devices.

The only aids we recommend for long-term use are those which promote good spinal posture or walking mechanics (e.g. back supports or shoe inserts like orthotics).

Chronic-pain sufferers develop *protective responses* to avoid pain. For example, a person with low-back and leg pain will limp to avoid putting weight on the painful side. As a result, the biomechanics of his walking will be distorted, and some muscles and joints from the foot up to the spine will be overstressed. At the same time, the muscles on the other side will weaken from underuse. This imbalance and stress gradually result in more pain.

Reconditioning Exercises

Regardless of why you've become de-conditioned, there are specific reconditioning exercises you can do. Exercising can have a positive effect on the muscles and on other soft tissues in the painful area. Properly exercising an area can reduce stiffness, strengthen muscles to help support the area, and increase blood flow. These results act to improve the functioning of the area and can reduce signals that are feeding into the pain system.

Exercise which has been properly designed by a physiotherapist or a physiatrist (rehabilitation-medicine specialist) can have a dramatic effect on a chronic-pain problem. One case in particular makes this clear. A young woman had suffered from low-back and leg pain for many years and had developed a chronic-pain syndrome. Our physiotherapist at the clinic discovered that the leg pain was partially due to pressure on the sciatic nerve. This problem could be relieved by a brief exercise routine that was effective in a remarkably short period of time. This exercise routine could be performed in a matter of minutes and it, along with other pain management strategies for her low back, allowed her to return to school on a full-time basis.

The imbalance that I discussed in the de-conditioning section is typical of what may have to be addressed in your exercise program. Too many people return to pre-injury levels of activity without taking into account that some muscles have to be strengthened more than others. This is because their exercise programs have not been individually designed and supervised by an expert in the field of rehabilitation.

For this reason, I will not set out any exercise programs in this book. *Every chronic-pain patient requires an individual program.* However, there are a few basic rules we have found quite useful in relieving chronic pain.

We have found that stretching and loosening exercises, rather than weight-lifting exercises are better at alleviating a chronic-pain condition. People whose pain results from tense muscles don't need to strengthen them any more — they are already strong. What they need to do is to reprogram them to be loose, supple, and relaxed.

My clinical experience has shown that a significant number of people obtain an analgesic effect from anxiolytic exercise done in moderation. We recommend swimming, cycling (both the stationary and outdoor kind), fast walking, rowing, low-impact aerobics, etc. The one exercise we tend to discourage is running or jogging, because there is often too much mechanical stress on the body. This stress can aggravate an existing weakness and eventually defeat a re-conditioning program by producing more pain than relief.

The bottom line when it comes to exercise programs is that a chronic-pain sufferer must have the help of an expert — such as a physiotherapist, physiatrist, or kinesiologist — when setting up a reconditioning program. If your exercise expert is unfamiliar with the special needs of a chronic-pain sufferer, either find one who is, or show him or her this book.

CHAPTER

8

Cognitions and Pain

~~~~~~~~~

What is cognition? *Cognition* is the process of thinking and knowing in the broadest sense, including perception, memory, judgment, and so on. It involves our thoughts and ideas, beliefs and attitudes. It encompasses the body of knowledge and the perceptions about the world that we accumulate in various ways throughout our lives.

I Think, Therefore I Hurt

In this chapter, I want to focus on the following facts and show you how important they are to chronic-pain management:

1. Many factors influence your cognitions about pain.
2. Your cognitions influence how much pain you feel.
3. You can change your cognitions, and therefore how much pain you feel.

Many things influence our cognitions about pain, including the beliefs our society holds about pain, our past experience, parental role models, the "meaning" of the pain, the context in which the pain occurs and our control over the pain experience.

Throughout the ages, various societies have interpreted the meaning of pain differently, with the result that the people in those societies learned to think about and respond to painful stimuli in specific ways. For instance, in many primitive societies, pain was associated with visitation by an evil spirit. In ancient Greece, pain was considered a challenge to be met with courage and stoicism, while in ancient China, pain was thought to result from an imbalance in male and female forces within the body (yin and yang). In the Judeo-Christian tradition, pain has been viewed as a punishment for sinful behavior and as having a redemptive quality. In modern western society, these notions have been largely replaced by the "disease model". As we have seen, this model has its own limitations.

On a more individual level, each person has his or her own particular cognitions about pain. *Those people whose cognitions lead them to react negatively are prone to developing chronic-pain syndrome. This is because cognitions alter the amount of pain we experience.* They do so by influencing the functioning of the central pain system, just as emotions and behavior do.

This is a difficult concept for many people to accept. Since we have been raised on the Descartes model of pain, there is no room in our thinking for the effect of cognitions. Descartes told us that pain travels in a straight line from the site of the injury to the brain. There is no room in this model for cognition. Indeed, we now know that cognitions have a profound effect on the amount of pain we feel, as the following examples will illustrate.

In Chapter 5, I related the story of the young soldier at Guadalcanal, and how he reacted to three separate "wounds". The first two times he *thought* he had been severely injured, and he experienced severe pain, though in fact he had sustained no more than a scratch. However, on the third occasion he felt no pain even though a leg was blown off. His anticipation of pain was more crucial to his experience of pain than the actual damage to his body was.

Dr. Beecher, who reported this case, also compared soldiers who had been wounded in combat to civilians who had sustained similar injuries in domestic or industrial accidents. He found that only one soldier in four asked for morphine after being wounded in battle, although none of the soldiers interviewed was in shock. The important fact was that the soldiers viewed their wounds as an escape from combat, and perhaps from death. They were almost euphoric at the idea of going home. Their attitude was one of relief, and to them the pain involved was insignificant compared to the prospect of dying in further combat.

Civilians with similar wounds reacted quite differently. The traumas dramatically affected their lives, and they experienced far greater pain on average than the wounded soldiers did. There was nothing "beneficial" about their injuries, and their negative thoughts caused them to perceive their pain more intensely.

Let me remind you of another way in which cognitions affect pain. I have already described the miraculous effect that placebos can have. Placebo-responders believe that they have been given painkilling medication, and that belief itself releases painkilling chemicals, namely endorphins. *The greater the patient's belief in the power of the medication, the greater the relief that person will obtain from the placebo*. Therefore, your belief in the effectiveness of a treatment and your belief in your ability to get better can actually help you achieve this goal. This is a self-fulfilling prophecy of the highest degree.

One of the oldest placebos pre-dates medicine itself. Faith healing presents a very dramatic example of the way in which belief can produce recovery. Although faith healing is "unscientific" and most people (including myself) are skeptical about its curative powers, there is a powerful placebo effect at work in people who believe in it. Through the release of endorphins, believers can experience some pain relief. So medicine does not have a monopoly on the placebo effect.

In many instances, people suffer lessened pain because of the meaning and a reward associated with the pain itself. The reward can be of a religious, personal, or societal nature. Many of you will recall the movie *A Man Called Horse*, in which an Englishman who chooses to become a warrior member of a North American Indian tribe goes through a rather gruesome ceremony to gain tribal membership. The pain experience produced by rites of this nature is reduced for several reasons. First, the participant *chooses* to take part in the rite; secondly, the rite has religious significance; and thirdly the person will be rewarded with acceptance by his peers after the ordeal has ended. For all these reasons, the pain becomes more manageable.

Another important element in cognition is that of self-control. People who are in control of a situation can experience less pain than those who feel powerless. For example, studies have shown that patients who have suffered severe burns and are forced to undergo the painful process of debridement (the removal of dead skin) are better able to tolerate the discomfort if they are allowed to perform the procedure themselves.

Another example of the role cognitions play in chronic pain is shown by the change in a person's attitude toward pain before and after a serious, perhaps even life-threatening, illness. Ray suffered from tension headaches off and on, like the rest of us. The pain was no big deal and he simply took some pain pills or relaxed. One day he got a headache that didn't go away quite as easily. The pain became so intense that he went to the hospital and the doctors diagnosed a brain tumor. They removed it and Ray made a complete recovery. Several months later, Ray had another headache. He immediately thought, "My God, the tumor's back!" This time the pain was just as great, which reinforced his fears, and he decided to go back to the hospital. His belief about headaches had now been changed by his experience with the tumor. But fortunately this headache was only caused by tension!

Ray had learned that headaches could be the signal of a life-threatening condition. Unless his perception of the problem reverts to what it was before the tumor, he may develop a chronic-pain problem.

All the above examples illustrate the importance of one's cognitions of pain. Cognitions can play a major role, especially in chronic pain. In order to reduce your pain, you have to alter your cognitions. *You must develop attitudes similar to those who have conquered their pain.* This process is called *cognitive restructuring*.

Cognitive Restructuring and Pain

Many people who develop a chronic-pain problem manage to cope with it very well. It does not disrupt their lives a great deal, and in time they find that their pain decreases in intensity. These people are called "copers". They have positive cognitions about pain. At the other end of the spectrum are "catastrophizers", who react in an entirely negative way to pain. Most of us fall somewhere in between these extremes.

If a person finds that chronic pain is controlling his life, he must restructure his cognitions. As you will soon see, you can analyze your negative cognitions to better understand them, and then take steps to replace them with more positive cognitions. A vital aspect of cognitive restructuring is a comprehensive evaluation of your *self-talk*.

You Don't Have to Be Crazy to Talk to Yourself

We all talk to ourselves, although we may not think of it as such. We have an internal self-monitoring system, an inner voice that helps us to monitor our actions and directs our activities to accomplish our goals. This is what psychologists call self-talk.

A few years ago, a baseball pitcher known affectionately as "The Bird" became a fan favourite, because he talked to himself, the ball, and anything else in his vicinity while he was pitching. This was his way of telling himself what to do and how to do it properly, and it worked well for him. All of

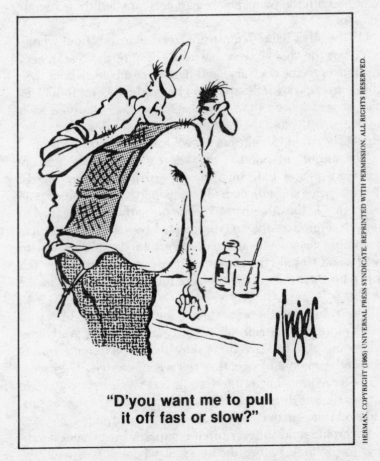

"D'you want me to pull it off fast or slow?"

The difference between "copers" and "catastrophizers"

us do the same thing, although usually less obviously. However, the things we tell ourselves are not always positive.

The disruptive effect of negative self-talk is shown in the results of a recent laboratory experiment. Volunteers were exposed to electric shock and researchers had them record their self-talk in response to the painful shocks. Some people told themselves that they would be fine once the testing was complete. They assured themselves that no harm would come from the shocks and they used strategies like distraction to cope with the pain. The researchers labelled these people "copers".

On the other hand, "catastrophizers" worried about whether or not the shocks were harmful (despite the researchers' assurances to the contrary) and they were anxious about their ability to cope with the shocks. They did not want to make a bad impression on the researchers, and they doubted their ability to withstand the fleeting instances of pain. They were obviously afraid, despite having volunteered for the project.

The important point is that the catastrophizers actually reported greater pain than the copers did. In other words, their negative self-talk actually magnified the amount of pain they felt. On the other hand, the copers in the test managed to actively minimize the amount of pain they felt. Rather than becoming negatively aroused, they told themselves not to worry and to take the testing in stride. As a result, they felt less pain than the catastrophizers did when exposed to the shocks.

The results of the experiment led researchers to try to teach more positive self-talk to the catastrophizers. And those who were able to learn these skills showed a definite reduction in the amount of pain they felt when retested. They were far less anxious during the testing and were better at techniques such as distraction. The results of this experiment provide vital clues in the battle to conquer chronic pain.

A chronic-pain sufferer often compares his present condition to the time before the accident when all was well. Patients frequently make statements like, "If only I hadn't had that accident, I would never have wound up like this. Before I got hurt I was perfectly healthy and pain-free. But not now."

This type of before-and-after comparison is futile as well as depressing, because the past cannot be changed. The clock cannot be turned back. This is destructive self-talk. What we teach our patients to do instead is to compare how they feel on a day-to-day or week-to-week basis. We want them to think about how they felt a few weeks ago, how it compares with their present state, and how they will feel in the future.

The major problem in changing self-talk patterns is that people are usually unaware that they have them in the first place. They have to learn to listen to that continuous self-talk and identify the catch phrases that can cause the trouble.

You can do this by writing down your self-talk. This is not particularly easy, because your self-talk patterns are often irregular and the thoughts can cover a wide spectrum. However, when it comes to chronic pain, certain catch phrases occur over and over again. Here are a few examples:

"I'm never going to get better."

"Why me?"

"What will people think of me now?"

"Why can't the doctors help me?"

"I must be going crazy!"

"What is really wrong with me? I must have some horrible, fatal disease."

"I just can't cope with this pain any longer. It's hopeless."

To make matters worse, this kind of self-talk usually occurs when the victim is at a crisis point, when he or she is more stressed than usual for any number of reasons. Even a "coper" can break down into negative self-talk under these conditions. It takes a lot of discipline and motivation at such times to write down in full one's self-talk, but it's important to do it if the negative messages are to be eliminated.

The second step is to review your self-talk notes in order to identify the negative thoughts you are expressing to yourself. A good way of making the most of this step is to look back the next day at what you have written down. It is easier to be objective after a period of time. You may also be somewhat surprised by what you see. "Did I really say all those negative things yesterday? No wonder I felt lousier as the day went on," you may say. This is a typical reaction when one reads notes some time after they were recorded.

Step three is the hardest part of the process, because it involves replacing negative self-talk with statements that tell you how to react positively and effectively. This step is vital; it is not sufficient merely to *stop* negative self-talk. The resulting void must be filled by *positive* self-talk. But it will take weeks or even months before your new positive self-talk becomes automatic.

We ask our patients to write out some sample positive self-talk messages, and then decide which ones they want to use to replace the negative ones. Since they are now listening carefully to every negative self-talk statement, we have them immediately and deliberately replace them with positive messages. For example, they may begin by asking themselves, "Why can't I be the way I was before I was hurt?", but they must immediately replace this with something like, "I'm better today than I was last week, and I'll feel even better next week."

I saw a woman in my office several months ago who had been involved in a serious car accident. Her belief systems were about as negative as possible, as was her self-talk. She was convinced that only bad things happened to bad people, and she proceeded to tell me the story of how her accident had happened.

She told me that she had been driving home from work one night when she came to the usual intersection in the road. This time, impulsively, she took the less common route instead of the usual one. She was hit by another car while on this road. Although the accident was not her fault, she castigated herself for her impulsiveness and "poor judgement". She also believed that the pain was "set" and that she had no control over herself or over it.

After some time, I was able to convince her that her guilt and self-criticism were a form of negative self-talk and we worked on changing both. She came to realize that she was not "bad" and bad things didn't always happen to her. She became aware that she did indeed have control over her actions, as was demonstrated by her ability to choose the different route home. She could also see that she was aggravating her pain problem by believing that she was being punished.

The more positive belief system that we helped her to develop conflicted with her old, negative beliefs and she gradually discarded the latter. She now leads a relatively normal life, and is much more at peace with herself and more optimistic about the future.

To summarize, let me emphasize that negative self-talk is an automatic process — a subconscious act. In order to replace it, you must first became aware of it. Once it is no longer subconscious, you must develop positive self-talk in order to replace it. In turn, the positive self-talk will have to be practiced for weeks or even months before it becomes so natural that you will do it subconsciously. This is not an overnight process!

Stop That Thought!

Often it is difficult for people to modify negative self-talk, because it frequently occurs at times of crisis. At such times, the negativity of your self-talk is overwhelming and comes upon you so quickly that you do not have time to react calmly and logically. This is when you can utilize a technique called *thought-stopping*.

Thought-stopping means using a very sharp command to yourself. You can use commands such as "Stop! I don't want to hear that any more", or "That's nonsense! You know better than that!" You can make up phrases that are most effective for you and remember to use them in conjunction with your replacement of positive self-talk. These will startle you out of your negativity and allow you to take better control of your thoughts. Thought-stopping is not a long-term solution to negative self-talk, but it can come in handy to break repetitive, destructive thinking.

Imagery: The Video Within

Not all self-talk is verbal. Some of it occurs in the form of pictures in our minds about the way we see ourselves and the way others see us. Some of these pictures are realistic, while others are symbolic representations that carry a special meaning for us. Imagery is simply another way for us to communicate with ourselves.

The uses of imagery are threefold:

1. to change your self-talk patterns;
2. to replace existing negative imagery;
3. to act as a pain-control strategy, by itself.

I will talk about the first two uses in this chapter, and the third will be discussed in Chapter 11.

Imagery is a useful way to change self-talk patterns. You can employ it by imagining difficult events that have happened in the past or may occur in the future and imagine yourself in each of these situations, applying your new self-talk skills. This rehearsing for the real situation is often best accomplished when you are in a relaxed state (see Chapter 10).

My clinical experience has shown that the most effective way to erase mental images is to replace them with other images. You can test this yourself by imagining that you are in an open field on a beautiful sunny day. The sky is bright blue, contrasting sharply with the green grass. A few fluffy clouds meander lazily overhead. On the crest of a nearby hill, you see a magnificent white stallion silhouetted against the blue sky. A gentle wind caresses the horse's mane and tail, making the animal look even more statuesque and regal. You are stunned by the beauty of the scene.

Now try to imagine the same scene without the stallion. The horse will continue to enter the picture no matter how hard you try to erase it from your memory. Suppose, however, you put something else in the stallion's place atop the hill — let us say an elephant. Just imagine this huge beast in the middle of your picture and you will find that the stallion is gone. One image has been replaced by another. Understanding the use of replacement imagery is crucial when it comes to changing your cognitions.

The Rocky Horror Picture Show

Many chronic-pain victims suffer from destructive negative images of themselves and of what bothers them. They often imagine the worst things going on inside their bodies when they are in distress. Many of my patients describe feeling knife stabs in their backs or corkscrews being pulled out of their spines.

One patient told me, sheepishly, that he found himself imagining that there was a gremlin swinging from a meat hook imbedded in his back. Whenever this poor fellow moved the wrong way or walked along, the gremlin's swinging made the meat hook rip up his lower back. The resulting pain was often so excruciating that the man would collapse to his knees.

"It even sits down with me at the dinner table when I am eating. I can't enjoy a meal any more," he told me.

I had a thought. I decided to encourage him to use imagery to counteract the negative picture he had in his mind. "Suppose you poison his food," I suggested half-jokingly. "That would get rid of him for good." The man took my advice, and several weeks later I was pleased to hear that this use of imagery helped him do away with his dinner companion.

The fact is that people tend to fear the worst when they are injured. I recall a time when I fell and damaged my rib cage. The pain was agonizing, and I had difficulty breathing. I was frightened, because I imagined a broken piece of rib jabbing into my side and perhaps piercing my lung. It was not until the doctor showed me the normal X-rays at the hospital that I began to feel better. Once reassured that there were no broken ribs, I immediately turned all my negative self-talk into positive self-talk. "I'm okay. I'll soon be better," I told myself, rather than "My God, what did I do to myself?" I no longer told myself to expect the worst. I knew that I would recover completely, and my anxiety and pain decreased right away. This knowledge did more for me than the pain pills the doctor prescribed.

My co-author has a friend who suffered from acute back and leg pain. "I've got this terrible pain shooting down my leg," he said, "and the doctor told me it was because my sciatic nerve was being pinched by my disc. I'm terribly afraid," he continued, "that if I move the wrong way I can make my disc cut right through my nerve, and then I would become a paraplegic."

This man had a destructive image of his spinal column. He said that he could "see" his "sharp" disc cutting through his sciatic nerve, and it was not until he was told that discs are not sharp and this could not happen that he began to feel better. What finally convinced him that he was in no danger of becoming a paraplegic was his own examination of a model of the spine and his opportunity to hear an expert explain why his disc could not sever the sciatic nerve.

These stories illustrate the serious consequences that negative images can have on acute pain. They are much more destructive in a chronic-pain situation when they are maintained for a long period of time. You should examine your thoughts for these images and be prepared to replace them with positive ones.

As with negative cognitions, you can go through the same steps to dispel negative images. First, obtain reassurance that your pain is not a sign of serious injury. Sometimes all it takes is to see a healthy X-ray, as in my case. But X-rays cannot show soft-tissue damage (to muscles, tendons, or ligaments) and you might have to be otherwise convinced that your injury is not serious. The proper assurance can come from experts who know how to illustrate and explain just what is wrong and how it can be corrected.

Some of our patients believe they have bad backs because of scar tissue which has formed in the painful area. Sometimes they have surmised this after comparing notes with someone else who has similar symptoms.

Whether or not the scar tissue is a problem for them, if they *believe* that it is, it will have a great impact on how they respond. They will have an image of the scar tissue as the source of their pain. The problem with this is that people believe that scars are permanent. It stands to reason that a person who believes that permanent scar tissue has formed in her spinal column and is inflicting back pain will also be plagued by negative imagery that will hinder her recovery.

What I try to do is shift the person's understanding of his condition to one that is more manageable. We explain that many people have scar tissue with no pain. Scar tissue may or may not be causing his pain. It doesn't matter, because you can't eradicate it. We do know that shortened and tense muscles cause pain. We point out to the patient that his problem involves her back muscles, which often tighten up, go into spasm, and cause great pain. Muscles are attached to bones by tendons, which are cords of strong tissue. When a tendon is too tight, it irritates the sensitive nerve fibers at the point where it attaches to the bone. The fibers emit signals that are fed into the pain system, causing severe pain.

We teach the patient to replace the image of scar tissue with the image of a knotted muscle. Why? Because that makes the problem solvable. Knots can be untied, and the person can learn to do so mentally.

We have the patient imagine that his muscles have knotted up like a sailor's rope, and then we tell him to visualize untying the knots strand by strand until the muscles are loose and comfortably stretched. Whenever he begins to feel his muscles tighten up, he imagines himself untying the knots. Eventually he will be able to unravel the strands long before his muscles go into spasm, and he will be well on his way to breaking the vicious circle of pain, fear, anxiety, and tension-induced pain.

Now he no longer imagines his back to be a mass of scar tissue; he envisions a basically healthy spinal column with easily flexible musculature. Moreover, he has stopped constantly telling himself that he is a sick person with an intractable problem.

Using Your Behavior to Change Your Mind

A few years ago, I saw a patient in his late forties who had suffered a heart attack, and who complained of chest pains whenever he did any physical activity. His doctor had reassured him that his pains were caused by the muscles in the chest wall — a fairly common occurrence in post-cardiac patients. His chest wall had become a "vulnerable" area after his heart attack, and whenever he felt stressed or worried those muscles tightened up and caused him pain.

The doctors told him that his cardiovascular system had returned to a reasonably healthy state and that he need not fear another heart attack every time he felt some pain in his chest. But the man remained unconvinced. He could not return to work. He considered himself disabled and adopted an invalid-like lifestyle — just waiting for the next attack. After about a year of this, he was referred to me.

I, too, tried to explain that his pains were not dangerous, and I cited his doctors' reports. "That's easy for you to say," he replied. "You can talk until you're blue in the face, but you can't understand how scared I get when the pains begin. I keep thinking I'm going to have another heart attack."

I have found that the best approach to take with this type of patient is to employ incompatible response strategies. These are based on a concept known to psychologists and others as *cognitive dissonance*.

Cognitive dissonance is a state of inner turmoil resulting from contradictions in a person's beliefs, or contradictions between one's beliefs and one's actual behavior. The contradictions create a state of discomfort in the person, who will then be motivated to resolve them, because nobody likes to live with constant inner turmoil.

Cognitive dissonance results whenever a person's actions are incompatible with his or her beliefs. Long before psychologists were invented, the Catholic Church utilized cognitive dissonance to convert those who were not "believers". The Church knew that, even if you did not have faith at the outset, if you behaved as if you did, eventually faith would follow. They set up a conflict between a person's belief system and his or her behavior, and more often than not, behavior won out, with the result that the person became a practicing Catholic. This technique has not been lost on other religious organizations which also practice cognitive dissonance to win converts. If cognitive dissonance can work in religion, it can work in the treatment of chronic pain.

Since our heart attack patient was not amenable to positive self-talk and imaging, the only way to change his behavior was to create cognitive dissonance. We had him start with slow walking that did not induce chest pain and had him slowly shape the activity. Eventually he reached a level of activity that produced a state of cognitive dissonance, because his belief that he was a sick man was being challenged by his own vigorous activity. In time he began to see himself as a healthy person. Within eight weeks he was *jogging* to my office. When I last saw him in the office, I asked how he felt about his heart condition. He replied, "I still have the pain sometimes, but it doesn't bother me as much as it did. After all, it's hard to see yourself dying of a heart attack when you're planning to jog home that night." The baseline, shaping, and pacing techniques had worked to perfection.

When introducing cognitive dissonance, the activity change does not necessary have to involve exercise. With one of my patients, the trick was to get her out of bed and back into the kitchen. This middle-aged woman had been injured in a car accident. When the pain refused to go away, she became totally sedentary, because everything she did hurt. Every morning her family helped her out of bed and downstairs into the living room, where they deposited her on a couch for the rest of the day. There were telephones at either end of the couch so that she did not have to move to take a call. At bedtime family members helped her back upstairs and into bed. This routine had gone on for months, and the woman had become a total invalid, although there was no evidence that this was necessary. She had developed a severe chronic-pain syndrome.

When the woman came to see me, I realized that she and her immediate family could not envision a way out of her chronic-pain dilemma. To begin with, I had to convince the family that she could indeed lead a fairly active life, and they agreed to let me set a baseline and start a shaping and pacing program for her.

Two vital pieces of information emerged from my first meeting with the woman and her family. For one thing, she could walk at least a few feet without increases in pain; secondly, she loved to cook.

We began by having the woman walk unaided from the couch as far as the kitchen. This was her baseline. Gradually, we got her to undertake some minor cooking tasks. A breakthrough came a few weeks later when her family came home one day to find that she had prepared one of her specialties for them. She had begun to abandon her invalid-like lifestyle.

As you can see, we did not take an invalid and make her into a marathon-runner. But we helped her return to a healthy lifestyle. She is an *active* person again, and she no longer sees herself as chronically sick. She was also helped by the fact that the people around her learned to think of her as a healthy person.

Your beliefs and cognitions about pain are very important in controlling pain. There are two main strategies for changing your beliefs about chronic pain. One way is to replace them with more positive ones; another way is to make systematic changes in your behavior to accomplish the same goal. If you want to maximize your recovery, you should try to employ both strategies simultaneously.

CHAPTER

9

The Body Language of Pain

There are many ways that pain sufferers stand out from the crowd. I have been observing people with chronic pain for years, and most of them exhibit certain mannerisms and behaviors which portray their distress. These pain behaviors can be grouped into several categories:

1. *Bracing*: supporting themselves, for example by grasping the arms of an armchair to support their back, or by the use of artificial supports;

2. *Guarding*: protecting a painful area by limping, etc.;

3. *Grimacing*: wincing, twitching, jerking, frowning, and other facial expressions of pain;

4. *Moaning*: groaning, sighing, and other audible expressions of pain;

5. *Rubbing*: and otherwise touching the painful area;

6. *Complaining*: verbalization of the pain experience

Let me give an example that I see all the time. A patient with severe chronic back pain is visiting my office for the first time. As she walks into my office, her face is contorted with pain, she grimaces and limps with every step. When she reaches her chair, she grasps the arms firmly and gingerly lowers herself into the seat. She then twists and turns in the chair in search of a comfortable position. But whatever comfort she finds soon dissipates and she squirms in the chair throughout the meeting, in search of new, less painful positions. At the end of the session, she again winces as she pushes herself out of the chair. As she departs, her movements are as stiff as they were when she entered.

This woman communicates her pain to the rest of the world as well as to herself. For the most part she will be unaware of these behaviors and unaware of their impact on others.

When I ask her if her pain behavior in any way reduces her pain, she will tell me that it brings, at most, fleeting relief. The fact is that most pain behavior is unnecessary. This statement may surprise you, because we expect to see it in those who are suffering. We think of it as an automatic response which is forced upon us by the pain. Although this might be true in cases of acute pain, most chronic-pain sufferers have a greater control over this pain behavior than they think they do.

When I first started treating chronic-pain sufferers ten years ago, I felt very sorry for these grimacing, limping people. Then I began to realize that they needed my help, not my sympathy. Once pain sufferers realize the implications of their unhealthy behavioral patterns, they usually make every effort to change, and are quite successful.

A person who has pain but who does not show it has a far greater chance of recovering completely or of coping with the problem than one who is an "exhibitionist". Why is this? Experts agree that openly exhibited pain directly influences the pain system and therefore affects the amount of pain experienced in the long run.

Think of it as if you were standing in front of a mirror and continuously expressing the pain you feel, either by speaking to yourself or by facial and body expressions. The longer you watch and listen to yourself, the more serious and hopeless your fate will seem and the more pain you will experience.

Part of our program is dedicated to making patients aware of their pain behavior so that they can reduce it. Once this happens, they have a much better chance of controlling their discomfort. Later in this chapter, I will show you ways to identify and change your pain behaviors. But first, there is another reason why it is important for you to make these changes.

The "Third Law" of Chronic Pain

Not only is chronic-pain behavior a problem for the sufferer, it also causes emotional and behavioral responses in those who come in contact with him. The sufferer interacts with others in ways that elicit certain responses. You can think of this cause-and-effect as a variation on Newton's third law of motion — for every action, there is a reaction. For the pain sufferer, these reactions in turn become part of the mix that feeds the pain system.

In this way, well-intentioned family members often make it difficult for those with a chronic-pain syndrome to improve. For this reason, we find it very helpful to include in a treatment program any concerned others, such as friends and family of the pain sufferer. People who are constantly interacting with the sufferer have to learn how to identify and deal with that person's pain behavior, and how to adapt their own patterns of behavior so as not to inadvertently make themselves part of the problem.

Let's compare the lifestyle and behavior of two people with the same degree of angina (caused by inadequate blood supply to the heart during exertion).

Person A displays little discomfort. He attempts to carry out his activities at work and at play as he did before his troubles began. Whatever adjustments he has made to his lifestyle because of his ailment are not drastic enough to produce a sedentary pattern of behavior.

Person B, on the other hand, shares his pain with all those around him. He complains about his discomfort and displays his feelings with a variety of mannerisms and facial expressions. He worries constantly about his health, either openly or to himself. He has developed a sedentary lifestyle, out of fear of attempting anything that might bring on anginal pain, which, he imagines, may be a precursor to a potentially fatal heart attack.

In short, he slowly sinks into invalid-like behavior and thinking. His family and friends fall into the same trap by being overly concerned about his needs and protective of his "frail" heart. They excuse him from normal activities, and thus encourage his passivity. If he lifts a finger to do something, his wife says, 'Don't do that, dear. You may bring on an angina attack. You just rest."

Angina-sufferer B displays his pain so well that his loved ones are forced to respond to it and so get caught up in the process. His entire circle of family and friends unwittingly reinforce his pain system. By their solicitous actions, they are actually confirming his own fears of how sick and disabled he is. Their reactions will only reinforce his belief that he has indeed become a perpetual prisoner of his condition.

It is not that angina-sufferer A ignored the seriousness of his condition. It is simply that he refused to allow it to unduly interfere with his enjoyment of life and the goals he had. He took the necessary precautions to avoid aggravating his condition, but he got on with life. Moreover, he did not allow his family and friends to get caught up with his health problems. In the long run, he is destined to fare much better than B.

Old Dogs, New Tricks

One way to conquer pain is to learn how to change ingrained

pain behaviors. Naturally, the first step in controlling these behaviors is to be aware of the times when you display them. We pay careful attention to the way our patients move and sit and we ask them to start taking note as well. If this kind of awareness is difficult for you, you can ask a family member to observe you as well. When the target behavior occurs, you can employ techniques similar to "thought-stopping" that we discussed last chapter. Remember to make the instruction to yourself powerful and meaningful.

Secondly, we recommend the use of incompatible response strategies to eliminate pain behaviors. This sounds more complicated than it is. Quite simply, you must learn a new behavior to replace the pain behavior.

One example of how this works comes from a recent case of mine. A young man who had experienced neck and back pain for over two years had developed a mannerism of shifting his neck, shoulders, or upper body. He did this about twice a minute, on average, and more often if he was feeling more pain. He said he was only vaguely aware of this behavior. He had started this body movement because he found that the shift briefly alleviated the pain. But after a short while it had become a habitual, repetitive pain behavior that was actually reinforcing the pain.

To treat this problem, we had him sit in a comfortable position for as long as he could without making the movement. At first, he could only do this for about two minutes. With this as the baseline, we cut it in half to one minute and then had him sit without such movements for an ever-increasing period of time (shaping). He increased the time by fifteen-second increments every two days and performed three such practice sessions per day. As he practiced the replacement behavior, he was getting his body used to what it felt like to sit normally. Over about ten weeks, he was able to increase the replacement behavior to ten minutes, and then it abruptly disappeared. Now it shows up only when he is under a lot of stress.

The second example is of a woman who needed gait-training. In other words, she needed to relearn the proper way of walking. Because of a back and hip problem, she favored her left leg, and she walked bent forward with a shuffling gait. As I mentioned in Chapter 7, this kind of distortion has an impact on the musculature, but it also has an impact on the person's self-image, on others around her, and ultimately, on the pain system. With the help of our physiotherapist, she learned how to take one normal, properly balanced step. Then we had her shape this behavior five times a day by walking ever-increasing distances. At first, she reverted easily to her gait-problem during the rest of the day, but soon the new walking habit replaced the old.

Not all pain behaviors involve physical mannerisms. The external props you use — crutches, canes, etc. — can also count as pain behaviors. As I mentioned earlier, these devices weaken some muscles but they also have a behavioral impact on pain. We caution our patients not to rely too much on such things as back rests or supports, even though some back supports such as the McKenzie Lumbar Roll or the Obus Forme are excellent for maintaining proper posture. You have to weigh the benefit each device gives you against the potential long-term impact on the way you and others see yourself (i.e. as a chronic-pain patient).

Asserting Yourself

Chronic-pain sufferers sometimes use their pain to avoid doing things. "I can't cut the grass today, honey, my back hurts" is a typical refrain. They find it handy to plead pain rather than admit the task is unappealing. This person actually does have pain but the pain is not the real reason he does not want to cut the grass; the real reason has more to do with the World Series game on television.

If you think you are "getting away" with this behavior, you're mistaken. The hidden cost is that it reinforces the pain system. You are using pain to gain short-term rewards, and thereby rewarding your pain.

Assertiveness is the antidote to the above problem. Instead of meekly accepting your lot in life, you can assert yourself to get what you want. Whether or not you were assertive before your pain condition began, it would be a wise move to learn how to be more forthright in stating your wants and needs. (I am not talking here about being *aggressive*, which I would consider excessive in many cases.)

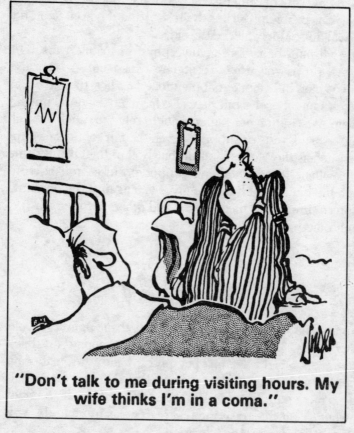

"Don't talk to me during visiting hours. My wife thinks I'm in a coma."

Malingering can serve many purposes.

Assertive behavior is positive and powerful without being overbearing. Assertive people have goals, definite needs, are optimistic about the future, and are more likely to take matters into their own hands than those with behavioral patterns associated with chronic-pain sufferers — such as negativism, passivity, fear, and inactivity.

I will admit that it is not easy to just snap your fingers and suddenly become assertive. But let me give you an example of a little trick that you can try when you are about to fall into an "excuse" trap.

Suppose your spouse suggests to you one fine evening that it would be nice to take in a movie, and she mentions a romantic tear-jerker she wants to see. You hate such films, so you immediately make an excuse to escape the torture.

"I can't go to the show, dear," you beg off, "my back is killing me. I'll never be able to sit through the movie."

"Oh, all right," she replies, "we'll just stay home and I'll find something on television to watch. Do you need a painkiller, or anything? How about a hot water bottle or heating pad?" Together, you have done a marvellous job of reinforcing your pain system.

What you ought to have done is said to your wife, "I'd like to go to the movies, but I don't think I could survive a soap opera. How about going to see that comedy I heard was so good?" Now what you have done is avoided being asked again to see the tear-jerker, and you have also avoided feeding your pain system. You have come out ahead by asserting yourself, without having upset her terribly. If you continue to respond in this manner when faced with unpleasant tasks or decisions, you will sidestep the trap of using pain as an excuse whenever it is convenient.

Making It Work!

By now, you should realize that I am advocating healthy

behavior to overcome pain. The epitome of healthy behavior in our society is being able to work.

For one thing, work is good for the psyche. It takes your mind off your woes and it makes you feel useful, which improves your self-esteem. You are better able to overcome your chronic-pain problem if you feel good about yourself. For another, any sort of activity, occupational or otherwise, helps break the pattern of invalid-like behavior.

But how do you get from being disabled, unemployed and out of the work force for many months or years, to performing a productive job that is psychologically and financially rewarding? That's quite a climb!

There are three stages to this process. You may not be able to participate in all three, but ideally, you would. The first stage is part-time volunteer work, then building up to job simulation and, finally, moving on to the workplace (part-time and then full-time).

The nice thing about volunteer work is that it's readily available, it's socially useful, and it puts you, the chronic-pain sufferer, into a work-like environment with little or no risk of failure. It is usually flexible, so you can start off with a few hours a day, if necessary. But you should built it into your schedule, so you don't fall into the trap of doing it only when you "feel like it". You commit yourself and you do it regardless of the level of your pain.

People tend to discount the importance of volunteer work because it's unpaid. That isn't the point. It's a stepping-stone to your eventual goal.

When a person has been disabled, but has a job to return to, we obtain the cooperation of the employer to set up a job-simulation program in the patient's home. Job simulation involves setting up equipment in the patient's residence and simulating work tasks. In this way, the patient can build stamina by performing tasks which will be required upon his or her return to the plant or office. For example, we have worked with a Ford employee whose job was to assemble brake parts. We obtained the parts from the plant and the man practiced the job at home.

On the first attempt, he was able to work for only two hours before experiencing a flare-up of neck pain. Here was a man who had to go to work eight hours a day. Had he gone right into the job full-time, he would have failed. So we used shaping and pacing. Over the next few weeks he was able to build his stamina up to six hours. At this point, he was ready to return to work. For the first three days, he needed permission from his boss to take time out when he felt pre-pain cues, but after this he had to take a full work load.

Six months after he had returned to work, I called to find out how he was doing. A new supervisor had been assigned two months earlier and when I asked him how Mr. P. was doing with his neck problem, he said, "What neck problem?" Mr. P. was doing fine and is continuing to do so four and a half years after his return.

The final goal in most cases is actual competitive employment which can be of a part-time nature to begin with. Ideally, you should have an opportunity to build up to full-time work in the same job, but if this isn't possible, it's still important to take the part-time position first. We have been able to apply this strategy to help people return to automotive assembly lines, construction jobs, truck-driving, baggage-handling, and clerical positions.

When you eventually make it back to full-time work, if you continue to experience pain on the job, there are other pain-control strategies you can apply to maintain your new level of functioning. We will now turn to a discussion of these.

CHAPTER

10

Relaxation and Pain Control

Imagine a television pitchman grabbing your attention with this spiel: "Is your body tired and your brain racing? Do you want relief? Well, my friend, step right up, lie down, and RELAX!"

A simple solution to a complex problem? Well, not exactly simple, but well worth the effort, because relaxation is like a mini-vacation. It is useful for combatting stress, pain, and a whole host of related conditions. Not only that, it is also perfectly harmless: the only side effects are pleasant — you might accidentally fall asleep.

When I use the term "relaxation", I mean much more than propping your feet up in front of the television after a hard day's work. I am referring to specific techniques that soothe the muscles and the nervous system and can reduce or eliminate pain. Relaxation is a state of meditative calm and peace that you will learn to recognize and welcome.

Taking a Break from Pain

There are three ways in which relaxation can help you to

overcome a pain condition. First, it helps control muscular tension, which is often associated with chronic pain. Secondly, it has a soothing effect on the nervous system by reducing arousal. Third, there is evidence that it releases endorphins, the body's natural painkillers.

In my experience, successful relaxation has both a short-term effect and a long-term effect. In the short term, it can greatly reduce pain; in some people it can completely eliminate pain while they are in a relaxed state. The long-term effect is more subtle; relaxation can reprogram the pain system to reduce pain over the long term. I think of relaxation sessions as producing a cumulative effect as they progressively undo the effects of all the stress and tension that have been in control of your chronic-pain problem for so long. Finally, relaxation can teach you to become aware of tightness and other sensations in your body, and this awareness can be used in other pain-control strategies.

Relaxation techniques are somewhat like the different types of meditation that we associate with the gurus of Eastern cultures. Almost all these techniques have certain features in common:

1. They are conducted in quiet, fairly dark surroundings with little stimulation present.
2. You will have something specific to focus on, not just visually, but mentally as well.
3. You achieve a calm state of mind.
4. Finally, you are not to be interrupted during the relaxed state.

Many professionals have training in relaxation techniques, including psychiatrists, psychologists, and other therapists. Several relaxation routines have been recorded on tape, and they are available on the market as self-help aids. Many of these tapes have excellent background music and sound effects, but, as I shall explain, they often fail to take into consideration the special needs of the chronic-pain sufferer.

I have seen some chronic-pain patients who doubt the usefulness of relaxation methods because of previous unsuccessful experiences. If I mention that part of our program includes relaxation techniques, they groan.

"I tried that stuff before," they say, "and it didn't work. Is that all there is?"

"Just a minute," I say. "How did you learn relaxation before?"

They might reply, "I got a tape to listen to. I couldn't really understand everything, but I tried really hard to relax. Anyway, the pain stayed just as bad, so I gave up after a couple of days."

Or I hear this: "I went to this meditation group. It was a couple of hours a night, twice a week. I felt great while I was there, but if I hurt a lot at home or at work, I couldn't do anything about it."

Another answer I often get is, "I was taught how to relax by a therapist. It was fine when I could do everything just as he told me — you know, dark room, absolute quiet, and all that. But when I'm at work and I do something that makes me hurt a lot, I can't just run off to a secluded room and meditate for half an hour. I'd lose my job."

As you can see from the above, simply being exposed to relaxation is not the solution to chronic pain. Let us examine these problems, beginning with the first response.

Not everybody can learn from a tape. Many people need personal attention — contact with a teacher — before they can properly understand what they are being told. Another problem with tapes is that they enable you to relax while listening, but they fail to teach you how to use the technique *as a pain-control strategy*. What do you do when you have a flare-up and your tape is not with you? The tape has probably not taught you how to deal with emergencies, or how to use relaxation techniques to prevent sudden attacks of severe pain.

A final problem with tapes is that I have seen patients become dependent on them, which means that they have come to need the tape to produce the pain relief. This defeats the flexible nature of relaxation and undermines your sense of control.

The second person has obviously not been taught to make use of what she has learned in group sessions away from the relaxing environment where her teacher holds forth. As with the person who had tried to learn how to relax with the aid of tapes, she is unable to cope with emergency situations and she has not been taught strategies to prevent a pain attack.

The third patient is in the same boat as the second. He has not learned the skills that will enable him to deal with a pain episode outside of a quiet, dark room and especially in a work environment. Moreover, his relaxation therapy has not been combined with physical therapy and other strategies which can help prevent work-related stress and physical injury to a vulnerable part of his body. This lack of a *multidimensional* treatment program is a problem most chronic-pain patients run into when they undergo relaxation therapy.

The Four Types of Relaxation

There are four basic types of relaxation. The first is called the Jacobson Technique, after its founder, Edmund Jacobson, a psychologist who advocated relaxation by alternatively relaxing and tensing various muscle groups.

The second is *autogenic relaxation*, which emphasizes concentrating on the bodily sensations of relaxation such as warmth, heaviness, tingling, etc. The third involves *imagery* techniques and the fourth is an *audio-focusing* approach, using a mantra (a word or phrase). For our purposes, the mantra could be a form of positive self-talk, such as, "Every day in every way I am feeling better and better." This last technique is useful for many people, but I prefer the other procedures.

I employ the other three techniques, singly or in various combinations, depending on the needs of an individual patient. Eventually you will be able to determine by yourself which the techniques, and combinations of them, works best for you. I will discuss visual imagery in detail in the following chapter, so we will focus here on the Jacobson and autogenic-relaxation techniques.

Learning How to Relax

If you are just beginning to learn to play the piano, you cannot expect to play a Beethoven sonata in the first session. The same is true of relaxation. Relaxation techniques are like other skills; they have to be learned and this takes time. Some people pick up the basic techniques fairly quickly — in a few sessions. Others require more time.

After I teach my patients how to relax, I have them practice the techniques on their own every day until they are comfortable and confident with what they have learned. Some require only one practice period a day, although three daily sessions are preferable.

When I begin teaching my patients how to use relaxation therapies for chronic-pain conditions, I let them know that they may feel various sensations in their bodies while relaxing — such as warmth, tingliness, drowsiness, heaviness, lightness, or floating. Not everybody experiences the same feelings while relaxing. Some people feel tingly and light; others may feel warm and heavy. This is not important. What matters is that the sensations make you feel comfortable and loose — at peace with the world and with yourself. These sensations are a signal that you are, in fact, relaxing. You should be soothed and calmed by such feelings, not frightened.

I also reassure patients that they are in control at all times, and that they have nothing to fear. Some people mistakenly associate relaxation with hypnotism and they believe that, under hypnosis, a person loses all control. They are wrong on both counts.

I stress to my patients that, in relaxation, I am simply their guide. Relaxation comes from within; a tape or an expert in person cannot *make* them relax. It is the inner state of mind that counts, not what their guide is telling them in soothing tones.

Many people try too hard to relax. I recall one of my patients who literally ordered his body to relax. This is like ordering yourself to fall asleep! It doesn't work! Naturally, it creates more stress than it relieves. Relaxation is a passive art — you have to just "let it happen".

Here are a few tricks that you can use to avoid interruptions during your relaxation sessions: take the phone off the hook, and inform those around you that you are not to be disturbed for at least thirty minutes. Go to a quiet place; that means no radio or television, or other such distractions.

Many people begin to relax, only to have negative thoughts intrude on their reverie. They find themselves worrying about something that has happened, or a chore that should be done immediately. Relaxation time is just that, and no more. If you think of something that must be done shortly, just tell yourself that it will be accomplished soon after your relaxation period has ended. If it's important, you won't forget about it.

I suggest using self-talk to tune out these thoughts and replace them with instructions such as "I'll think about that later". Or you could use visual imagery, such as imagining yourself literally putting these thoughts aside, into a place of safekeeping, until you can turn your attention to them.

Another technique is to write out all the tasks and troubling thoughts before you do your relaxation routine and then place the piece of paper out of sight. Writing down the problems helps you to articulate them and put them into perspective. Since you have already finished noting them and you aren't worried about forgetting them, you can now turn to the task of relaxing your body.

You might feel guilty about taking time off to relax. You might consider it "goofing off". You should dispense with this idea immediately. Those of you with chronic pain absolutely require relaxation periods! You are following a carefully devised program when you take these relaxation periods. You are not being lazy! If you wish, you may think of the time as being spent reprogramming your body, much like programming a computer. *This time is not wasted*.

An Ounce of Prevention

I have found that relaxation can reduce pain under many circumstances. However, once you are in the midst of a severe pain episode, it is less likely to be effective. The point is to be able to recognize when a pain episode is coming on, so that you can avert the episode altogether. If you have learned to become aware of your body, and some of the pre-pain signals that precede the onset of a pain episode, you can use all of your relaxation skills to prevent the onset of more pain.

In relaxation, it is common to become drowsy. But you are not to fall asleep during daytime relaxation for two reasons. First, the relaxation period is a time to *consciously* deal with a pain problem. Secondly, if you do fall asleep, you will upset your normal sleep patterns. As you will learn in Chapter 14, sleeping outside of normal nighttime hours can disturb your sleeping pattern.

There are various ways of staying awake during a relaxation period, but the most reliable is to use an alarm clock, which you can set to go off in about a half hour. This way, even if you doze off, you will not be asleep long enough to upset your proper nighttime sleeping pattern. I use the thirty-minute period, because most people take about twenty minutes to totally relax their bodies and need another ten minutes or so in that totally relaxed state.

Another way to help keep yourself awake is to give yourself a suggestion beforehand that you are to use the time to relax only, not to take a nap. Whenever you begin to feel drowsy during your relaxation period, the suggestion acts as a reminder to remain awake.

Deep Breathing

The way we breathe is a reflection of our physiological state. We all know that if we become anxious or engage in exercise, our breathing is automatically affected. What we do in relaxation is reverse the normal order of events. We teach people how to deliberately change the way they breathe in order to induce a physiological state conducive to achieving deep relaxation.

Breathing opens the door to relaxation in another way. It not only prepares you for a state of relaxation, but is relaxing in itself. Deep breathing can also serve as a cue; it reminds you to relax. Once you begin to associate taking deep breaths with feeling relaxed, you can learn to start breathing deeply at the first indication of a pain episode. This, in turn, triggers a relaxation state which will help you prevent the pain.

Take a moment now to practice the art of deep breathing. Close your eyes and slowly exhale through your mouth. When you have no air left to expel, slowly begin to inhale through your nose until your lungs are full of fresh air. Hold this air in your lungs until you feel slightly uncomfortable. Then repeat the exhaling procedure. When you are exhaling, you will literally feel the tension draining out of your body.

Deep breathing must be done *slowly*. The most common error that people make in deep breathing is doing it too quickly. Take it slow and easy. Otherwise, you run the risk of hyperventilating and may even pass out.

Setting the Stage

In the relaxation procedure I am going to take you through, I will ask you to focus your attention on the various sensations throughout your body, particularly when you tense up compared to when you relax. You are *slowly* going to relax one part of your body at a time. It would be helpful if you look at Figure 11 before you start. This diagram will help you visualize the muscle groups you will be working with.

One more thing before I take you through a combined Jacobson and autogenic technique. I have found that certain chronic-pain sufferers can experience a temporary elevation of pain in a particular area if they strongly tense that area. If this happens to you, you should tense the area only slightly or simply focus on the autogenic suggestions of warmth and heaviness when relaxing that part of your body.

Now that you have some facts about relaxation, let's get started. You should first get comfortable in a quiet room where you will not be disturbed. I suggest you remove your shoes and find a position in a chair or on a couch that provides you with as much relief from pain as possible. Is whatever you are resting on — a chair, couch, or bed — fully supporting your weight? If you have a back or neck problem, are you sure that your position will not cause you pain in a few minutes, thereby interfering with your relaxation period? You will probably feel and concentrate better if your eyes are closed, but you may keep them open if this puts you more at ease.

FIGURE 11   *Main Muscle Groups*

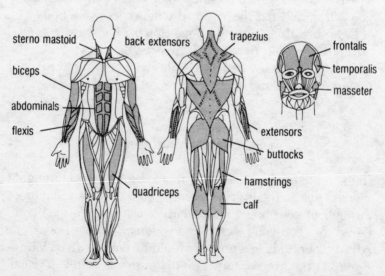

sterno mastoid

back extensors

trapezius

frontalis

biceps

temporalis

masseter

abdominals

flexis

extensors

buttocks

quadriceps

hamstrings

calf

Now dim the lights and start into the first stage of relaxation — deep breathing. Take five or six deep breaths, as I described above. You have now started to relax.

We will begin muscle relaxation with your right arm and hand. Hold that arm out stiffly and clench your fist, until you feel tension, tightness, and a slight discomfort. Then release your arm; it doesn't matter if you do this slowly or quickly. Let it rest, fully supported on the bed or chair. Keep concentrating on that arm. You may feel some residual sensations of tightness in the arm, but it will soon become relaxed and loose.

Turn your attention to the fingers of your right hand. Let them dangle freely from the end of your hand. You might feel some tingling and warmth and heaviness. These sensations are signs of relaxation. Continue to concentrate on these pleasant feelings.

Now that your fingers are totally relaxed, I want you to imagine these same sensations slowly moving into your hand and up your arm until you feel them all the way up to your shoulder.

Once you have finished with your right hand and arm, repeat the process with your left hand. Continue to concentrate on how different it feels to be totally relaxed compared to being tense.

When both your arms are completely relaxed, you can move up to your shoulders. To tense your shoulders, raise them as high as you can without hurting. Feel how tense they are. Then let them drop, and notice how they slowly begin to feel as pleasantly relaxed as your arms. Savor the feeling for a moment, and then move on to the neck.

The muscles in the neck are often taut for the same reasons as the shoulders, so this session ought to make them feel much better. In order to first tighten the neck muscles, you can press your head back against whatever is supporting it. Then slowly release the tension and feel the neck muscles slacken. They may become warm and tingly; they will certainly feel relaxed and comfortable. Concentrate on these pleasant sensations.

Once your neck is fully relaxed, you can move on to the facial muscles, which in most of us are often tensed although we don't realize it. This tension causes headaches and facial and jaw pain. The areas easiest to work on are the forehead, the area around the eyes, and the jaw muscles. Let's begin with the forehead. Raise your eyebrows as high as you can while keeping your eyes closed. Then slowly allow the muscles in the area to relax. You should experience the same sensations you have already felt in the other relaxed parts of your body.

Next, clench your teeth, but do not grind them. Now slowly relax the jaw muscles. Don't worry about your mouth hanging open a little; you are relaxing, not posing for a picture. Notice how relaxed your whole upper body now feels. You may even feel as if you are floating. Continue to concentrate on how pleasant the sensations are, particularly compared to the feelings of tension.

Turn your attention to your legs and feet. Raise your right leg. Point your toes and curl them downwards. At the same time, tighten your calf muscle and the back of your thigh. Then let your leg and foot relax and drop back to a comfortable position. As you did with your fingers and arms, concentrate on the pleasant sensations you are now enjoying in your toes and then allow the same sensations to gradually work up through your foot and leg. Repeat the procedure with your left leg and foot.

We have now reached the torso. I want you to pay particular attention to your abdominal muscles first. Take a medium-sized breath and hold it. Tighten your stomach muscles until you feel the tension there. Then let those muscles relax and slowly exhale.

Your entire body should now feel warm, loose, and relaxed. Take the next few minutes to savor this new feeling. Turn your attention to various parts of your body and sample them to make sure that they are all feeling warm, heavy, and loose. If any area is not yet relaxed, repeat the tensing procedure in that place. You may be experiencing a sinking or floating sensation, which is perfectly normal.

Now that you have gone through the first relaxation session, you will want to practice this technique between one and three times a day until you feel comfortable with it. I do not want you to try using relaxation yet to control pain or fall asleep, because at this point you are still developing skills.

Shaping Relaxation Skills

Once you have mastered the basics, you can gradually shape your new skills to maximize their usefulness. You cannot always be at home when pain occurs, so you must learn how to adapt your skills so that they can be applied in different situations. In a work environment, you will likely have to sit in your chair in a noisy, well-lit area, with only five or ten minutes in which to relax. You have to learn to control a pain experience *by yourself* whenever the situation arises and without the benefit of a tape recording or a quiet, dark room.

Let me give you two examples of how people can use their relaxation techniques to advantage in situations over which they do not have complete control.

One of my patients suffered a severe whiplash injury in a car accident. After this happened, she was very nervous and tense whenever she drove, because she had vivid memories of the accident. With our help, she learned how to relax while in the car. We taught her to make use of spare moments at a stoplight or in a traffic jam to relax her neck muscles. Rather than letting her neck muscles stay tense from the stress, she envisaged them unknotting and relaxing. These techniques helped her to keep her pain at a very manageable level even while she was in her car.

Another patient worked on an assembly line. His chronic-pain problem was not directly related to his work, but the constant stress of performing the same tasks over and over caused him considerable discomfort a good deal of the time. We discovered that he had become quite adept and quick at his task, so he had a few seconds between each installation. With our help, he learned how to use that precious time to relax. Consequently he is now able to get through a normal work shift without any serious pain problems. For this man, mastering this pain-control strategy made the whole difference between being able to keep his job and having to quit and live off disability payments.

These patients achieved these remarkable skills by starting with basic relaxation and then shaping their ability so it could be applied in a specific situation.

How can you learn to do this too? Start by practicing the basic routine that I have set out and then, once you are comfortable with that, change the situation slightly. For example, you might do one of the following as a first step: turn on the overhead light, or open the door and let a radio play in the next room, or sit up in a comfortable chair. Practice relaxing in the new situation until you are comfortable. Then take another step which might include turning on the television or opening your eyes, and so on. The idea is to approximate the conditions of the environment in which you wish to be able to use the relaxation strategy. The shaping steps that you follow should be determined by the goal you wish to reach.

Variations on the Relaxation Theme

I will discuss two variations which may enhance the effectiveness of relaxation in your particular case. These are the use of relaxation cues, and combining relaxation with exercise.

In addition to shaping your relaxation skills to meet your needs, you can also develop relaxation cues which can bring on a relaxation state quickly under various circumstances.

The cue that you choose can be one of any number of things, including deep breathing, a phrase like "Take it easy", a visual image, a particular word, or any other signal that you choose to develop. The key to making a cue work is to consistently use it at the same time that you are practicing relaxation. This pairing of the two activities creates a strong association so that, over time, the cue itself will be enough to make you relax. You can use the cue in circumstances when you cannot conduct a full relaxation.

Relaxation and stretching exercises can be used together. Relaxation helps to release tension in muscles and stretching exercises can augment this release. In some cases patients have found that it is best to do the exercises first and then follow them up with a relaxation period. Others report that starting with relaxation and following with the exercises is the best. I suggest that you experiment with these two options to see which way works for you. You might also want to try yoga or t'ai chi which are combinations of the two disciplines.

EMG *Biofeedback*

Some people have a problem relaxing a specific painful area of their bodies. They need another tool to help them shape their relaxation skills — the *biofeedback* device.

EMG (Electromyographic) biofeedback is a way of measuring muscle tension in specific parts of the body. Muscles release small electrical impulses which are picked up by electrodes on the skin. Tense muscles produce strong electrical impulses which are interpreted by the device, and then played back to the individual in the form of an auditory or visual cue — such as a beep or a blip on a screen. The feedback tells people if they are tensing up a muscle group, or are successfully relaxing the muscles. The biofeedback itself is not doing anything to them; it is simply teaching them how to recognize when muscles are tense and how to recognize when they have relaxed them. In that way, it helps them control their pain.

Many of our patients have had great success with biofeedback devices. We often provide a machine for home use so the patient can use it as soon as he or she senses the onset of a pain episode. The technique is painless and the machines are battery-powered so there is no chance of an electrical shock. The machine measures your electrical impulses, but produ-

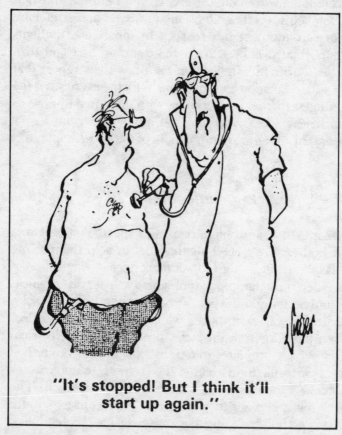

"It's stopped! But I think it'll start up again."

Biofeedback!

ces none of its own. To use biofeedback, you simply tape the electrodes to the skin of the painful area for about thirty minutes, once a day.

You will need help in obtaining this type of device and learning how to use it. Most cities have private biofeedback clinics or hospitals where machines can be used. Just remember that it is a teaching tool that you will use only temporarily until you have learned to successfully relax the tensed muscles yourself.

Finally, relaxation is also an important stepping-stone to learning the related techniques of imagery and self-hypnosis, to which we will now turn.

CHAPTER

11

Imagery and Self-Hypnosis

There are two other major pain-control techniques available, and their effectiveness is limited only by your imagination. I am referring to imagery and self-hypnosis. Like relaxation, these techniques release endorphins and affect the functioning of the pain system over both the short- and the long-term. Some people will be able to learn the techniques by reading this chapter, while others will require assistance from professionals. Both groups will benefit greatly from their efforts.

Imagine, if You Will ...

Imagery techniques start with relaxation as a base and build from there. You should go through the same preliminary steps to set the stage as you would for relaxation, but instead of focusing on muscle tightness you focus on developing images for your mind's eye.

Imagery involves visualizing and focusing on events or places that are completely absorbing. The image is usually a picture, but can also include the other senses, like hearing (perhaps music or surf), smell (salt air, flowers), and tactile sensations (a breeze). In fact, the more senses you can call into play, the more vivid and absorbing the image will be. One highly successful technique is to replay familiar scenes in your life that you have found very pleasant and enjoyable, particularly events that took place before your chronic-pain problem began. Childhood events or scenes often have warm emotional associations that make them very absorbing.

There are three major types of visual imagery that can be used to fight chronic pain. The most common one is called *distraction*; it is the easiest technique to learn and the simplest to apply.

Distraction

Distraction is a form of escapism. To start off, we want you to feel warm and comfortable — similar to the sensations you experienced with the autogenic relaxation technique in the last chapter. You are to concentrate fully on this pleasant sensation, totally eliminating any thought of your pain and other problems from your mind.

Think of where you would most like to be. For many people that place is a beach, perhaps recreated from your last vacation. So we shall try to create a scenario that will make you feel warm, cozy, and relaxed. The scene need not be one where you have been before; it can be from a movie or a painting, or you can even create the scene from an imaginary perfect world.

To help get you started, I will create a scene for you from my last vacation. You are lying on a beautiful beach, soaking up the warm, gentle rays of the sun. The sand is white and clean, and its warmth soothes your body, making you feel at peace with the world. The temperature and humidity are right where you want them, so that you feel neither too hot nor too cool. You hear the rhythmic lapping of waves on the shore, and the gentle rustling of leaves on nearby trees. You smell the invigorating, fresh sea air. Somewhere in the distance is the faint sound of pleasing music.

Concentrate on all those sensations that please you so much. You feel as if you are in heaven, because you are so relaxed and content. Pain that you may have been experiencing before you began your fantastic escape will become insignificant. You will want to replay this scene whenever you begin to experience the onset of a pain episode.

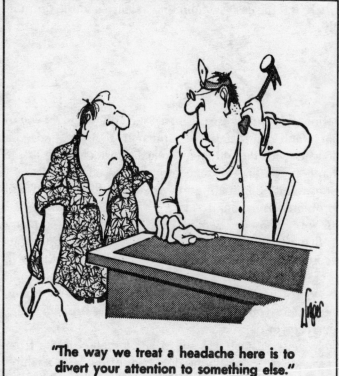

"The way we treat a headache here is to divert your attention to something else."

The fine art of distraction.

Of course, you may not be a beach lover. If so, you have to imagine other scenes that you find pleasant. If you love brisk mountain air and the pristine beauty of uninhabited peaks, you can replace the beach with your favorite mountain retreat. Some people prefer to return to scenes from their childhood, when life was simple, happy, and pain-free. It doesn't matter where or how far back you go, as long as the scenes remove you from the here and now.

Focusing

The second type of imagery you can use for pain management is called *focusing*. This technique will probably require more practise, but it can be a very useful tool if conducted properly.

Instead of departing from the here and now, you will focus on the problem at hand. You are going to concentrate on your pain so that you can take steps to reduce it.

Many of you probably spend a good deal of your mental energy trying *not* to focus on your pain. Perhaps when you focus on your pain and dwell on it, you can feel it begin to increase. You may fear it will trigger an episode of severe pain. The way to overcome this fear is to understand that if you can use focusing to make your pain worse, *you also have the power to make it better*.

In the last chapter, I mentioned the image of untying knotted muscles. This is an example of focusing. In this case, let us imagine your painful back muscles are very tense, perhaps even in spasm. Concentrate on those muscles; imagine them tied up tightly in knots. Focus on the end of one muscle and then begin untying the knot at that point, until the entire muscle is unravelled. Repeat the procedure until you feel that all the muscles in the area have been unknotted. You will know when you have succeeded by the fact that your pain has lessened and the area feels less tense.

Another approach is to imagine your pain in such a way that you can reduce it in a series of gradual stages or steps, going from high to low. Another common method involves the use of colors. Let us say you have a very painful shoulder. Concentrate on that area, and imagine the sore spot as being bright glaring red. Now imagine that color gradually changing, as a rainbow does, to dull red, then orange, yellow, green, blue, and finally purple. As the color becomes progressively cooler, the painful area also "cools down" and the discomfort decreases. When that color has turned to its coolest shade, the pain will be insignificant.

Yet another way of using the focusing technique is to move pain from one location to another, and eventually to move it out of the body altogether. Let's take that painful shoulder of yours. Once again, while concentrating on that area of your body, you focus on that pain slowly spreading from your shoulder down into your upper arm. Once you have this established, move the pain again, this time into your forearm. Repeat the process until you have the pain firmly trapped in your fingers. Now, imagine the pain slowly seeping out the tips of your fingers and into thin air. Now you feel it, now you don't. You have eliminated the pain from your body. This technique is very effective once it is mastered through practice.

Re-labelling

The third imagery technique is called *re-labelling*. It is called re-labelling because, whether you know it or not, you have *already* labelled your pain to begin with. You probably think of it "as if there's a vise around my head," or "as if there's a red hot poker stabbing my back," or "it's like there are needles sticking into my head," or "as if there's a corkscrew in my side," and so on. In other words, we play this "as if" game with ourselves without even thinking about it. We label our pain as a way of describing it to ourselves and others.

By now you know that this type of imagery can be very destructive and can increase the amount of pain you feel. Would you be willing to put a little energy and creativity into re-labelling your pain if you knew that you could use these labels to actually reduce your pain? This is the goal of re-labelling.

Take each of the examples I have used and see if you can take control of them to change your pain. For example, while you are in a relaxed state, think of that vise around your head and imagine a hand gradually undoing the clamp and thereby relieving the pressure. Or change the red hot poker into a thermostatically-controlled wand and imagine yourself gradually turning down the heat step by step.

Perhaps the "needles" can be turned into acupuncture needles (which hurt very little; see Chapter 16). Imagine the electrical current to the needles gradually being turned up and the pulsations slowly drowning out the sensation of pain. Eventually there is nothing left except the tingling of the electrical current.

By now the principle should be clear: first adapt your pain label to something that you can modify and then imagine yourself taking control of that stimulus. Take your time and build in as many details as possible. The more details there are, the greater the effect. Try inventing new labels for your pain that are less frightening and less threatening and practice modifying them as well. The possibilities here are limited only by time and your imagination.

Self-Hypnosis

There is a very fuzzy line marking the distinction between imagery techniques and self-hypnosis, and I do not wish to try and clarify that distinction now. Let me just say that hypnosis seems to be a slightly deeper form of relaxation than imagery and that there are elements of *suggestion* — both during and after hypnosis (post-hypnotic suggestion) — that are not present in imagery.

Self-hypnosis is nothing more than hypnosis a person does by him- or herself. This is a deep state of relaxation that can be achieved by many people after practise. Not everyone is capable of reaching this level of trance, but everyone can benefit from learning the imagery that I describe in the next few pages.

There are various ways of achieving an hypnotic state. You can begin by starting a relaxation procedure — you lie down, take a few deep breaths, use your relaxation routine, etc. until you reach your normal level of trance. Concentrate on techniques that take you to the deepest state of relaxation that is possible for you. The deeper the relaxation, the more suggestible you will be; and the more suggestible you are, the more you will be able to modify your pain levels.

Imagery is involved in hypnosis, of course. But, while you are visualizing a particular scene, you are also giving yourself suggestions for pain reduction. Here are two common examples.

You have achieved a deep state of relaxation. Now, in your mind's eye, you are going to stand at an easel and draw an outline of your body. Now, take red paint and brush it over the areas where you hurt the most. Then use orange paint for the parts of your body that hurt only a little. Once you are finished, imagine taking a pail of whitewash and pouring it over the outline of your body. Watch the whitewash gradually wash out the reds and oranges of your pain.

Now, imagine yourself beginning to back away from the outline of your body and watch as the picture begins to get smaller. Keep going until the picture is the size of a postage stamp. Imagine a strong guest of wind coming along and blowing the picture off the easel. It flies through the air and lands on the back of your head. You then lock that picture into your mind, because on it there are no pain spots. Keep that whitewashed picture for future reference, because you can recall it whenever you begin to feel a pain episode occurring.

If colors don't work well for you, try this method. You have been under a tremendous amount of stress, and your headaches have returned, along with persistent neck and shoulder pains. Imagine yourself sitting in a chair. Beside you on the floor is a bucket of powerful anesthetic. Stick your hand into the bucket and keep it there until it is fully anesthetized. It will feel as your mouth and face do when the dentist injects novocaine into your gums.

Then take that hand and place it on your throbbing head. Imagine the anesthetic seeping into the pores of your forehead. Feel the numbness and tingling sensation gradually spreading to your head until it is as anesthetized as your hand. Soon your headache diminishes to the point where it no longer bothers you. Move your anesthetized hand to your neck and your shoulders. As the anesthetic flows from your hand to these areas, the pain slowly decreases and eventually becomes insignificant.

Just relax for a few moments and notice how good you feel. You have numbed the pain with the anesthetic from the bucket. Whenever you feel the onset of a pain episode you will want to repeat this image in your mind. Perhaps, with time and practise, all you will require is the touch of your hand to the painful areas.

Putting It All Together

Now that you have learned the basic skills and strategies of cognitive-behavioral therapy, you can begin to apply them to managing and controlling some of the pain-triggers that I discussed earlier in this book. These triggers include emotions, personality, analgesic use, and sleep. Once you have these pain-triggers under control, you will have all the skills necessary to overcome chronic pain.

CHAPTER

12

Chronic Pain and Emotions

~~~~~~~

The clock strikes 3 A.M. You have been sleeping restlessly, and now you've been awakened by sharp pain caused by your tossing and turning. No matter how hard you try, you cannot get comfortable. The pain becomes more severe, and you are unable to fall asleep again. Because everyone else in the house is fast asleep, you have no one with whom to commiserate. You do not want to wake up anyone else to seek solace or help. You don't want to take any more medication than you have already taken during the last twenty-four hours. You feel frustrated, angry, despondent. You get out of bed and head for another part of the house where you can suffer alone or find some sort of relief.

What sort of havoc has been wreaked upon your emotions by this episode, which has occurred all too frequently over the past few weeks or months? How does this psychological wear and tear contribute to your pain problem? In this chapter we will take a closer look at the relationship between pain and emotions and how you can influence this relationship to control your pain.

What are the emotions most commonly associated with pain? If the pain is acute, we might experience fear, anxiety, and even panic. This is because the onset of sudden pain may signal a severe, even life-threatening, situation. Can the sudden acute pain in the chest area be owing to a heart attack? Are the pains following an accident indicative of a potentially fatal or crippling injury? These are the fears commonly felt in such circumstances.

However, if we are dealing with chronic pain, the emotions are somewhat different and generally less intense. The most common emotions associated with chronic-pain conditions are frustration, anxiety, anger, depression, and, in extreme cases, despondency. Chronic-pain sufferers are not afraid they are going to die; they fear not being able to cope with the present or the future. They begin to doubt that they will ever be able to live normally again, and they develop emotional states that actually feed that doubt.

Depression

The most common emotion associated with chronic pain is depression. Depression is more than simply feeling sad or "down" for a few days. It seriously interferes with many of the enjoyable aspects of life — social activities, laughter, sexual enjoyment, work satisfaction, and so on. It has generalized effects on appetite, sleeping, sexual desires, memory, concentration, the speed of movement, and fatigue. Depressed people have trouble seeing the light at the end of the tunnel. They have difficulty motivating themselves to do things and they always manage to see the black side of a situation.

As you know, chronic-pain sufferers begin to lose control over their lives and see no way of changing their fate. You lose hope, and once you have lost hope, you are likely unable to take steps to reverse the situation, even if a solution is presented to you. There have been several studies that illustrate why it is that these experiences produce depression.

In one experiment, dogs were subjected to electrical shocks. One group of animals were warned that the shocks were coming by the sound of a buzzer. The other group received no warnings at all, and were zapped at random intervals. Those dogs who had warning of the shocks coped reasonably well with the pain, which they demonstrated by their relatively "normal" behavior. The dogs who could not predict when they were going to be zapped exhibited quite disturbed behavior.

Similarly, chronic-pain sufferers often become despondent, because they can never predict when they will be hit by a pain episode. My patients often tell me that one of the worst aspects about their pain problem is never being able to predict when it will flare up. They spend a lot of their energy dreading the worst. Those who are better able to predict when and how they will experience pain are better able to handle the problem and to take steps to overcome it.

Another experiment involved dogs who were exposed to electrical shocks on a repeated basis. One group of dogs were exposed to a series of shocks which they could not predict or avoid. At first, every time they were shocked, they howled and tried to escape, but they couldn't. After several hours of this treatment, they became passive, lying in the cage and whining quietly whenever the shock was administered.

Then these same dogs were placed in a new cage in which they could avoid shocks by climbing up onto a platform. The experimenters taught the dogs how to avoid the shocks. Yet, whenever shocks were given, they failed to climb up onto the platforms to avoid pain. They had become too apathetic and depressed by that time to take any action whatsoever.

A second group of dogs who had not had the previous experience with the unavoidable shocks were also placed in cages with platforms. These dogs regularly used the platform to escape the shocks, because they knew early on in the experiment that there was hope for them if they escaped to the platform, and they did so.

The first group of dogs had developed a condition called *learned helplessness*. They had become too depressed from the earlier uncontrollable shocks to act positively in the cage with the platform. They had learned that their behavior had no effect on the pain, so they became apathetic and passive, even in a situation they *could* control.

These experiments help us to better understand the relationship between pain and emotional states. They indicate that chronic-pain sufferers will be less bothered by depression if their pain has some predictability and if they learn soon enough how to avoid it. The element of control is crucial in avoiding learned helplessness. If sufferers are unable to achieve some sense of control, they may become terribly depressed, occasionally to the point of utter despondency.

At this point it is necessary to stress again the crucial links between emotions and pain sensations. As we indicated in an earlier chapter, beliefs and expectations (that is, "mental states") directly affect the amount of pain or distress felt. Obviously, the opposite is also true: pain affects the emotions, "the way you feel". This two-way cause-and-effect flow is mediated by *neurochemicals* in the brain.

Now add one more element. You also know from previous chapters that physical activity can cause changes in the body's balance of hormones and neurochemicals. Thus it is apparent that all these physiological and emotional states form a tightly-knit web: physical activity, cognitions, and moods all affect each of the other states through changes in the body's chemical balances, and changes in the body's chemical balances determine to a large extent how much or how little pain you feel.

This interlocking unity helps to explain why cognitive-behavioral therapy works. In order to reduce pain and depression, the neurochemical balances must be altered. This can be done by administering drugs — and that is a common treatment. But that same result can *also* be achieved by changes in behavior and cognitions.

Treating Depression

Anti-depressant medication works fine for a certain group of chronic-pain sufferers, but it is not a cure-all. If you have not had a trial of anti-depressant medication, it may be worthwhile doing so. Find a doctor who knows how to prescribe these medications for chronic-pain management, because not all physicians are familiar with this. Usually, your physician will have you start off with a very low dose and work up slowly, until you are taking as much as you can tolerate. But anti-depressant medication has many side effects that are not well tolerated by many people.

I have found that anti-depressant medication and cognitive-behavioral therapy can work together well. Cognitive-behavioral therapy can do everything that anti-depressant medication can, and do it without side effects. You might achieve a more marked effect if you combine the two treatments.

Cognitive-behavioral therapy alters the neurochemical imbalances in the body, as the following study demonstrates. A group of patients who had been hospitalized for their depression were persuaded to be active and energetic for one day. The researchers did everything they could to help the patients forget their depression by organizing all sorts of events, including a Ping-Pong tournament and a party. In contrast to their normal lethargy and passivity, the patients agreed to take part in a wide variety of physical activities to keep them occupied throughout the day.

Their chemical levels were measured in the morning and at the end of the day. The second reading of these levels was much higher and the volunteers reported themselves to be — and appeared to be — much less depressed. In just one day the behavioral changes were enough to produce chemical and mood changes.

Most of us observe changes in our mood when we do something we enjoy to help us forget events that have depressed us during the day. For example, how often have you gone shopping after an exasperating day at work, or played an invigorating game of squash or tennis? Didn't you feel much better afterwards? Just imagine what you could do if you extended this routine into many weeks.

Since what we are talking about are behavioral strategies, you should apply the behavioral techniques of shaping, pacing, and anxiolytic activity (which are discussed in Chapter 7) when carrying them out. They will help you to avoid exceeding your tolerance level and will increase your stamina.

You can also use cognitive strategies to overcome illogical and self-defeating beliefs for which depression is a breeding ground. Since chronic-pain victims reach a point where they cannot see the light at the end of the tunnel, their self-talk becomes so negative that they convince themselves that life has always been a "downer" and they will never be happy again. All of this self-talk can be approached and modified by the strategies I outlined in Chapter 10. Using these cognitive strategies in conjunction with the behavioral strategies is the most powerful way that I know to break depression.

Anxiety

Anxiety is usually seen in the earlier stages of chronic pain. Instead of saying that life is no longer worth living, an anxious pain victim will engage in anxious self-talk, such as, "Will I ever be the same again?", or "Why am I not getting better faster?" Unlike those who are too depressed to react, chronic-pain patients who are extremely anxious behave like nervous cats up a tree about to be chopped down. They haven't quite given up hope, but they fear the future.

Anxious chronic-pain patients often exhibit pressured and rapid speech patterns. They have a host of nervous mannerisms of which they may not even be aware. One patient who suffered from frequent headaches came into my office, sat down, and immediately began rocking the chair (it was not a rocking chair) from front to back and side to side. He took out a wad of business cards at one point and shuffled them on my desk. Then he proceeded to make *me* nervous by straightening the papers on my desk. This went on for the entire half-hour session. And yet, when I asked how he would describe himself, he used terms like "calm", "cool", and "coper".

"How do you think your wife sees you?" I asked him.

"Well," he admitted, "she thinks I'm a nervous wreck. But she's nuts."

"Well, I tend to agree with her," I said.

"I was a navigator in World War Two," he told me. "When I first began flying missions over Germany, I was nervous as hell. But I managed to control my anxiety, and I still do."

I suggested to him that rather than controlling his anxieties he was ignoring them. Instead of dealing with the fears he had about his pain condition, he was sweeping them under the rug. Because of that, he had a tremendous amount of tension inside him, which was contributing to his pain condition. He had to learn how his pain system operated in order to come to grips with his problem, and he could not overcome the pain unless he started dealing with his fears.

"There will come a time when you will no longer be able to ignore your anxieties and your fears," I told him.

Unfortunately, he still could not understand my point of view. He thought I was saying that his pain was imaginary, even though I was telling him it was real, but aggravated greatly by his anxiety. He walked out of my office, and I have not seen him since.

He was typical of those who fail to recognize their own anxieties. One way to overcome this difficulty is to record your feelings as you self-monitor and then go back over them at the end of the week. Another way is to listen to those around you and ask them how they see you. Perhaps they are hesitant to speak up because they fear upsetting you. But if you ask for help, most people are all too willing to give it.

Anxious people who suffer from chronic pain often believe

that their anxiety will disappear once they get rid of their pain. They say, "I didn't have this anxiety before the pain started, so it is the pain that is causing it. All I have to do is get rid of the pain, and the anxiety will go away." As with other emotional states, the connection between anxiety and chronic pain is a two-way street. In other words, one way to overcome chronic pain is *first* to take steps to reduce the anxiety. You cannot wait until the pain goes away and hope that the anxiety will go away, too, because the anxiety is part of the pain problem.

You may also be using your pain as a reason not to make changes about which you are anxious — such as changing jobs or leaving an unhappy relationship. It could well be that your job or your spouse is contributing to your discomfort, and that you would feel a lot better if you made some changes.

I once treated a young woman who came from a southern European culture which was quite rigid and traditional. When she was sixteen she had married an older man, and consequently she had never learned to be independent. She had poor coping skills and was very immature for her twenty-two years.

When she was twenty, she had been injured in a car accident. As a result, her sexual, social, and recreational activities had come to a halt. She and her husband had drifted apart, and it was obvious that he was having affairs, but she was afraid to acknowledge his infidelity and confront him.

All her fears and anxieties were fueling her pain system, which had raised her discomfort levels far beyond what might have been expected with the type of injuries she suffered from the accident. In fact, her pain was the only thing that was holding their marriage together, since her husband felt guilty about his thoughts of leaving her, and she used his guilt to hold him to her.

What she needed most to do to reduce her pain was to reduce the level of anxiety in her life. To do this, she would have to confront her husband about his infidelity and take the chance that the marriage might end. However, this was impossible for her to do as she was overwhelmed by that possibility, which would mean that she would have to live alone and take care of herself. I could only suggest that she come back for therapy when she had dealt with the source of the anxiety in her life, for which she perhaps needed other types of counselling.

There are effective cognitive-behavioral strategies to deal with anxious patients who *are* in a position to take the necessary steps. We use the relaxation techniques as described in Chapter 10, and the anxiolytic activities set out in Chapter 7. We also delve into the causes of the patients' anxieties and fears so that they can understand the origins of them, and how they can be overcome. I recommend that you take the same steps if anxiety is a problem for you.

Anger

Anger is an exhausting and exceedingly destructive emotion. It fuels the pain system rather than dousing the flames. The type of anger that I am referring to is not just a fleeting outburst triggered by a minor irritation or an argument that is soon forgotten and smoothed over. I am talking about the kind of anger that constantly seethes below the surface, anger that produces almost uncontrollable rage in a flash and becomes an all-consuming passion.

Chronic-pain victims become angry for a variety of reasons. They may be angry with the pain itself, with health-care providers who are unable to help them, with the person who caused their accident, with those in their lives who do not understand their problems, or who refuse to sympathize with them, who ask too many "how do you feel?" questions, or who try too much to help. Their irritability, frustration, and anger are part and parcel of their pain experience.

They are particularly frustrated, because they are not able to enjoy the lifestyle they pursued before their problems began. Their lives become a series of compromises dictated by their pain. They can no longer go to a movie or a party, so they lie at home and watch television programs they don't even like. If their anger is directed at someone, that person becomes a focus for their thoughts and they relive the incident and imagine scenarios of revenge.

One patient with revenge on his mind had been injured while trying to assist a female co-worker when she was being harassed by a drunk. For his efforts, the drunk rewarded him with a solid punch to the jaw, which left him with chronic neck and jaw pain. Company management decided to sweep the entire incident under the rug.

Because the employee was insured by Worker's Compensation, he was unable to take legal action against the drunk. This made him extremely angry, both with management and the drunk. By this time he had traced the drunk to his home. He decided to avenge himself and he even bought a gun. He learned that the drunk was a wealthy man who owned a large estate with horses. My patient played with the idea of either "kneecapping" the drunk, or wounding one of his prize steeds. All this time his own pain problem became more severe; the anger was inflaming his pain system. Fortunately, he was sent to me before he mustered up the courage to gun down the drunk or his horse.

I immediately put him on a program of anxiolytic exercise and relaxation therapy. At the same time I helped him to examine and understand and thereby dissipate his anger. He used self-talk strategies as well as thought-stopping. Five months later he was back at work; he no longer sought revenge, and his pain had become insignificant.

Phobias

A *phobia* is an unreasonable fear that interferes with normal functioning in the phobic situation. The fear is persistent and anxiety attacks may be triggered in that particular situation. Why are we talking about phobias? Phobias produce a host of other negative emotions, such as anxiety and depression, which in turn may lead to more pain. Phobias can result from the same types of trauma that trigger pain conditions. People who suffer from chronic pain often become fearful of the events surrounding the accident and develop a phobia.

I have seen many patients who have developed driving phobias following motor-vehicle accidents. They become so fearful of another accident that they avoid driving whenever possible. In more severe cases, they may actually have anxiety attacks when they attempt to drive a car. If they are able to drive, the anxiety associated with driving can be a major factor in increasing their pain.

Fortunately, driving phobias are relatively easy to treat. The most common approach is called *systematic desensitization*. Systematic desensitization combines relaxation and imagery techniques in an interesting way. The first step is to imagine scenes associated with driving, and to rank them in order of the fear and anxiety they evoke. For example, the most fearful scene might be driving your car at the time of the accident. The least threatening scene might be picking up the car keys on your way out of the house. In-between are thoughts involving driving on a busy freeway and on a lonely country road.

Once the ranking has been established, you should get yourself into a relaxed state. Now, you start out by visualizing the least threatening scene. Picture yourself picking up your car keys and heading out to the car. If this scene makes you anxious, blot it out and return to a state of relaxation. Once you feel comfortable again, run through the same scene once more. After a few tries, you will be able to run through this scene without any anxiety.

You are now ready to proceed to stage two. Once again, return to a state of relaxation. When you feel comfortable, imagine yourself getting into the car but not actually starting the engine. As with the first scene, if you experience unpleasant emotions, return to a state of relaxation and then try again. Then imagine starting the car, and so on. This procedure is repeated until you can imagine yourself actually driving your car without any anxiety.

At this point, you are ready to go out into the real world and run through these actions in real life. This is the time to start using cues such as relaxing phrases or deep breathing, and so on to relax yourself as soon as you feel the onset of anxiety in the car.

One patient of mine, a flight attendant, was injured during a flight and developed a phobia about flying because of the accident. She had had the misfortune of being in a galley area when the plane hit unexpected turbulence. She had been thrown up and out of her seat and had hit her head on the roof of the galley.

The accident left her with severe head and neck injuries, which led to a chronic-pain condition. We were asked to help treat her pain problems, which we did. Although she did not express any direct fear of airplanes, it soon became apparent that she had developed a flying phobia. She began to realize that she could not get back onto an airplane.

We led her through systematic desensitization, as described above. In her case, one stage of treatment was to have her enter an airplane that was just sitting on the ground. (We had the full cooperation of her employer.) Eventually, she could imagine herself as a passenger on a plane, and she did in fact take a few flights as a passenger just to prove to herself that her phobia was under control. She is now back at work and has not suffered any relapses.

Humor

Humor is the flip side of the emotions usually associated with chronic pain. It seems fairly logical that if negative emotions can adversely affect the pain system, the opposite is also true — i.e. positive emotions reduce pain. What can be more positive than a few hearty laughs (assuming that they are not at someone else's expense)? If you are skeptical about this argument, I suggest you read Norman Cousins' book, *The Anatomy of an Illness*, which describes how he used humor to overcome a painful disease.

I often ask my patients on their first visit if they have had a good laugh lately. About eighty per cent of them say no. Yet the overwhelming majority would say that they used to have a good sense of humor before the onset of their miseries. They have come to see the darker side of life and have lost their sense of humor. If they can be shown the lighter side again, they will be far less likely to morbidly accept their lot in life.

Our experience has been that as our patients begin to regain their sense of humor, they begin to feel better. In fact, I can tell they are improving just by hearing them begin to make jokes about their condition and by their renewed ability to smile. Very few of them smile at our first meeting (I do not think it has anything to do with me); most of them are able to enjoy a good laugh after a few weeks of treatment.

How do we help our patients regain their sense of humor? First of all, everyone associated with our clinic must have a good sense of humor. And it tends to rub off. (Have you noticed how dour so many health-care providers seem to be? It is no mere coincidence that I decided to fill this book with "Herman" cartoons.) Secondly, we work with our patients to help them remember what used to make them laugh before their troubles began. Norman Cousins got together all the old movies that ever made him laugh and watched them when he felt down. Since he eventually recovered, in his case, laughter certainly proved to be the best medicine.

I don't want you to get the impression that all chronic pain can be miraculously cured by laughter. However, humor is a positive emotion, and such feelings do alter neurochemical imbalances. If you can enjoy yourself and even laugh at your own predicament, then those around you will respond in kind and you will develop a self-reinforcing positive cycle that will propel you toward recovery.

CHAPTER
13

Pain, Personality, and Intellect

Personality refers to the distinctive characteristics and response patterns that a person typically exhibits. We might note that a person is always optimistic, or always focuses on details, or is suspicious of others. A knowledge of someone's personality is what will help you to predict what he or she will do in a given situation. In general personality traits are evident at an early age and tend to change very little throughout a person's life.

Some social scientists believe that personality is inherited and that particular environmental factors only bring out traits that are already there. Other experts are more inclined to believe that environment plays the major role in shaping personality. I stand firmly in the middle. While I agree that some personality traits remain fairly constant, regardless of events and environment, other traits are shaped by traumatic occurrences, such as illnesses or accidents. Also, a series of events or exposure to a hostile environment can make for certain personality changes. So the old saying that leopards don't change their spots is not entirely correct.

There is at least one study that indicates that chronic pain can produce changes in personality characteristics. For many years psychologists have known that those suffering from chronic pain share certain personality traits that show up on tests like the Minnesota Multiphasic Personality Inventory (MMPI). Frequently these patients show tendencies to be depressed, to overreact to stimuli, and to be overly concerned about their health and their bodies.

These findings raise the question of whether or not there is such a thing as a *pain-prone personality*. That is, did these personality traits exist *before* the chronic-pain problems began, or did the constant pain cause the personality traits? In other words, do certain people suffer from chronic pain *because* their personality predisposes them to it, or does the chronic pain shape the personality?

In order to tackle this chicken-and-egg question, researchers looked at those chronic-pain sufferers who later obtained relief from their pain, either through surgery or other means. They found that the personality traits we just discussed disappeared after the pain was relieved. Once the pain was no longer a problem, these people were no longer hysterical, depressed, or morbidly concerned about their health.

There are two important conclusions that we can draw from this study. First, chronic pain can cause personality changes. This is important for those of you who have noticed changes in yourself. And perhaps others have made comments that "you are not the same person that I used to know." This is worrisome for many chronic-pain sufferers who do not fully comprehend what is happening to them. Personality changes such as impatience and pessimism can be very worrying. And we now know about the negative impact that worry can have on pain. I hope that this information will put you more at ease with the changes you have noticed in yourself. Rest assured that, as you gain more control over your pain and your situation, these changes will gradually fade and the old "you" will reassert itself.

The finding that the personality traits disappeared when

the chronic pain went away indicate that the traits on the MMPI were the *result* of the chronic pain, not the cause. The obvious conclusion from this is that there is very little evidence for such a thing as a pain-prone personality.

This understanding is also helpful to chronic-pain sufferers who might sometimes think, "Is this pain the result of something I did? Is it because of some flaw in my character? Have I got only myself to blame?" In my opinion, chronic pain is *not* the fault of the sufferer. On the other hand, since no one else can feel your pain and no one can take it away, the *responsibility for recovery* does rest with you.

This does not mean that certain characteristics cannot make you more vulnerable to developing a chronic-pain syndrome. In addition there are certain traits that make the *recovery* from chronic pain more difficult. For these two reasons it is crucial for us to take a look at certain personality characteristics that exacerbate chronic pain and to discuss strategies for modifying them. This chapter will look at how personality influences the treatment of chronic pain, and how, by recognizing some of your own traits in the examples I give, you can take steps to modify them.

The Over-Achiever

Perhaps the most common group of patients I see fall into the category known as *Type-A Personality*. People in this group are highly stressed individuals who place very high demands on themselves and must always be busy doing something useful. As a result, they often bite off more than they can chew, which means that they are regularly behind schedule. They are success- and achievement-oriented, and they tend to be obsessive about details. Since they are usually uptight and anxious, they have a difficult time relaxing and resting. They are apparently more susceptible to cardiovascular disease and stress-related illnesses.

Such people cannot cope with any diminished performance on their part. They also tend to place little value on small gains. For both these reasons, it is tremendously difficult for them to cope with chronic pain, which usually improves incrementally and leaves its victims with less chance of accomplishing superhuman deeds. Type-A people compare themselves with what they were like before their illness or accident, and when they realize they cannot measure up to previous standards, they become frustrated and anxious. Of course, this response only heightens their stress levels, which in turn aggravate their pain problems.

I have previously given examples of two chronic-pain sufferers with Type-A personalities: the business executive who went back to work too soon and tried to do too much, and the man who tried so hard to relax he became even more tense. In a typical situation, a Type-A person will notice that his chronic pain eases if he rests a few hours or days. But during the waiting period he becomes increasingly frustrated by his inactivity. This type of person becomes angry about not getting better immediately and believes that, in order to recover, he must push himself.

So he suddenly decides to re-attack his job or exercise program with a vengeance. He rushes out and undertakes a strenuous chore, like chopping wood, until the pain becomes so severe that he must rest again for a few days to recuperate from this act of madness. However, it is not all doom and gloom for these people; they can be helped.

Actually, I always enjoy treating Type-A people, because they are highly motivated to succeed. They are usually well-organized, they learn quickly and are willing to restructure their lives. And restructure they must. They have to learn not to try so hard. They must not demand past performance levels from themselves, and instead must become present- and future-oriented. They cannot expect to compete with their former selves, so they must adopt realistic new goals and new strategies that will offer them every chance of fulfillment in the future.

In addition, they have to learn to accept small gains, which in time will more than equal the "big bang" they have constantly sought for gratification. Most importantly, Type-A persons have to learn how to relax — to stop occasionally to smell the roses. Once they have learned this skill, the rest should gradually fall into place.

Shrinking Violets

When I think of this next group of chronic-pain sufferers, I am reminded of some of the fragile heroines in the plays of Tennessee Williams who are unable to withstand the ill winds of stressful situations. These are people who just do not land on their feet. They have poor abilities to cope and to take control of a situation. They tend to be passive when they should take charge and they let events overwhelm them.

Often they sail through life unscathed, until some traumatic event leaves them totally devastated. All of a sudden they come "unglued", because they are unprepared for adversity and don't know how to cope with it. When they fall victim to an accident or illness, their vulnerability leaves them in total chaos. Most of them have never been confronted with their own mortality — especially if they are young — and they have never had to cope with serious illness, either on their own or in loved ones.

One young patient of mine was involved in a rear-end collision. His car struck the rear of a truck and the truck gate broke off on impact. It literally sliced through my patient's windshield, barely missing his head. He had almost been decapitated. The event caused tremendous stress and trauma, and he began to relive the accident regularly. He was soon suffering from a *post-traumatic stress disorder* which combined constant neck and head pain with recurring nightmares, leaving him a veritable "basket case." He was in such poor shape that there was little I could do to help. He required psychiatric care, and I referred him to someone better acquainted with this type of problem.

Not all patients in his category are as difficult to treat. But this type of patient must now learn the coping skills that others take for granted. Inability to deal with stressful events points up their need to learn stress-management skills. They often respond well when they learn to readjust their expectations of life.

The Disaster Areas

Just as there are people who cannot cope with sudden distress because they have always sailed in calm waters, so there are those who are so used to stormy seas they are willing to accept constant pain as another fact of life.

Some of my patients have gone through a history of illness, family problems, and other traumatic stressors. Many were the children of broken, often violent, homes. Whatever nasty events had happened to them in their younger days had helped to shape their personalities. They have become used to suffering, and they accept it needlessly. Sometimes I get the impression that it is almost welcomed, because it is such a familiar condition of existence.

One young woman I saw was a single mother living in a dingy apartment in a shopping plaza. She came from wealthy parents but her childhood had been unhappy. She could not stand her parents and visited them only occasionally for the sake of her daughter. She and her daughter went to stay with her ex-husband on weekends, even though this time was punctuated with arguments and failed attempts at reconciliation. Within this context her neck pain was just one more problem, and the energy she had to devote to it was not sufficient to have an impact. The pain problem was not a high enough priority for her, because the rest of her life was in such a shambles.

People like this often do not respond well to therapy directed solely at their pain, and they may require intensive long-term counselling to help them resolve long-standing emotional and personality problems. They may benefit from cognitive-behavioral relaxation and exercise, but they are often unable to incorporate lifestyle and cognitive strategies into their situation.

Occasionally I see a patient whose spouse is also suffering from a pain condition, or other disorder. In such a situation, the pain and illness become a disturbing but ever-present part of their relationship. The constant level of disruption in their environment helps to maintain the chronic-pain state. In addition, if one spouse begins to improve while the other does not, there will be changes in their relationship, and this may cause the other spouse to undermine recovery.

In a case such as this, we have no choice but to treat the couple as a unit. The mutual support and understanding between the spouses can be an important component of any pain-management program.

Understanding Is the Key

We try to assess the personality traits of all our patients in order to find out what approaches could best help them overcome their problems. We can then concentrate on behavioral changes and cognitive strategies that are best suited to their own needs. And we are better able to figure out which relaxation and other strategies they can use to help them relax and change their attitudes about their lifestyles and goals.

Finally, I want to touch briefly on a major myth about chronic pain and personality types. As I mentioned above, I cannot identify one particular pain-prone personality. However, many people have the misconception that the typical chronic-pain sufferer is a lazy lout only interested in a free ride. He or she is often seen as a malingerer in search of a huge insurance settlement. When I began treating chronic-pain victims, I pondered these ideas. But my questions were soon answered. Very few of the patients I have seen over the years could be classified as malingerers. And my clinical experience seems to be quite similar to that of other pain-treatment specialists.

In my experience, there is no single chronic-pain stereotype. The one common factor is that my patients all experience pain, and have been in distress for at least six months. Otherwise they come from all walks of life, and from different ethnic, religious, physical, and social environments, and belong to both sexes and various age groups. Most importantly, they are all individuals.

This raises an interesting question. Is there, then, a group of persons with personality traits that enable them to *avoid* chronic-pain problems? I do not have an answer, although I suspect that some people naturally respond to an episode of pain with the same calm and methodical approach that I am advocating. Thus, they would be able to take steps to prevent themselves from succumbing to chronic pain. If we could only study them, I am sure that all of us would learn a lot.

Chronic Pain and Intellectual Functioning

A seldom-mentioned aspect of chronic pain is its effect on intellectual functioning — thinking and memory. People with chronic pain often complain of poor memory, clouded thinking, and an inability to concentrate on a task at hand. These changes have been confirmed by psychological testing. Understandably, they become alarmed and frustrated with themselves. They believe they are losing their intellectual capacities, and they are also fearful that the loss may be permanent.

Many well-educated chronic-pain sufferers have told me that they will read a newspaper and not remember any of its contents a few minutes later. Others report that they have trouble recalling events from one day to the next. Some are unable to concentrate long enough to work, or cannot collect their thoughts or express themselves clearly enough to hold a job. While these may be symptoms of depression or anxiety, they are also consistent with chronic-pain disorders.

The intellectual deficits associated with chronic pain are often blamed on analgesics, tranquilizers, and sleeping pills the person may be taking. While these drugs certainly play a major role, many chronic-pain sufferers who do not take any drugs display the same symptoms. I suspect that chronic pain alone is sufficient to cause at least some of these problems.

There are at least two possible reasons why chronic pain has these effects. First, it is feasible that neurochemical changes associated with chronic pain may be affecting a person's thought processes. There is much research to be done in this area, so this remains only a theory at present. Secondly, chronic pain drains mental energy from its victims, who are constantly focusing on their pain and on coping with it. They worry about their futures being destroyed by their pain condition. They expend enormous amounts of energy trying to cope on a day-to-day basis. The anxiety and depression associated with chronic pain syndrome can disrupt concentration and creative thinking.

Some of these problems can be treated using cognitive-behavioral therapy, although memory deficiencies may not always be totally recovered. If you have this type of problem, I advise you to keep a date book or diary handy so that you will have a record of your commitments. This will help you to avoid the embarrassment associated with memory loss.

As you begin to recover from your chronic-pain condition and concentrate less on your discomfort, you should gradually recover most, if not all, of your intellectual prowess. This renewed capacity in itself will make you feel better about yourself and help you improve your emotional state.

CHAPTER

14

Sleeping with Chronic Pain: A Bed of Thorns

〰〰〰〰

Sleep patterns are another important piece of the chronic-pain puzzle. Most people are aware of the fact that pain can disturb normal sleeping patterns. But not many realize that the converse is also true: sleep disturbances can also cause pain. This is one of the most overlooked aspects of chronic-pain management. In this chapter I will look at the relationship between pain and sleep, and suggest how some of these problems can be corrected.

The vast majority of chronic-pain sufferers I have seen have reported some type of sleep disturbance. Yet they failed to recognize how their pain problem was aggravated by sleeping difficulties. How do sleep disturbances cause pain and what does this mean for the pain sufferer?

Sleeping Beauty Never Felt like THIS!

In the 1970s a Toronto psychiatrist by the name of Dr. Harvey Muldofsky did some very important research on the relationship between sleep and pain. It had been noted before that many patients with chronic pain didn't feel rested in the morning, and reported feeling stiff and achy. Dr. Muldofsky was directing a sleep lab at that time, and he decided to look more closely at the sleeping patterns of these people by measuring their brain waves as they slept.

He discovered pain sufferers exhibited a particular disturbance in Stage Three sleep. (This is one of the four stages of sleep, ranging from light sleep to dreaming.) These patients did not remember having their sleep disrupted, but each morning they would complain of pain and stiffness. Moreover, the sleep was not refreshing, so they would awake feeling fatigued.

Up to this point, it was safe to assume that the pain was causing disturbed sleep and the patients were not getting all the rest they needed. But Dr. Muldofsky took this research one step further. He decided to take healthy volunteers with *no* pain problems and deprive them of normal sleep patterns by waking them at the point that Stage Three sleep began in the night. This had the effect of depriving these volunteers of Stage Three sleep just like the chronic-pain sufferers.

After just one night of this sleep interruption, the volunteers began to report pain, tenderness, stiffness, and other discomforts all over their bodies. They appeared to be developing the beginning stages of a pain problem and their complaints were similar to the complaints of the chronic-pain patients. The distress of the volunteers lasted until they were allowed to return to normal sleep patterns. This very striking and startling finding shows that a particular kind of sleep disturbance for even one night can cause pain. It demonstrates the crucial role of sleep in chronic pain.

The importance of this study is emphasized by my own clinical experience with chronic-pain sufferers. I have observed how overall fatigue levels can make pain worse as well as make it more difficult to cope with. In fact, our patients frequently note this relationship when they fill in their self-monitoring booklets. The effect of fatigue on pain over and above the loss of the sleep itself is a second reason for the need to control sleep patterns.

The Wide-Awake Blues

If pain is not a problem for you and you are otherwise content, you will find that you go to bed relaxed, comfortable, and tired, and fall asleep fairly quickly, perhaps within thirty minutes. Because this pattern has been going on for many years, your nervous system has developed the habit of quickly falling asleep. This is a learned association. But if there is an accident or the onset of an illness, you can quickly develop disturbed sleep, because you might turn the wrong way during the night and aggravate the pain, which in turn wakes you up.

Now you go to bed, toss and turn uncomfortably, and worry. Going to bed is now an opportunity to worry about your condition, because it is easier to focus on your discomfort in the dark. It is all too easy to dwell on your health and the problems that have resulted. Perhaps you replay the accident in your mind or focus on your future. This additional stress, in turn, compounds your discomfort.

Another complicating factor is that chronic-pain victims are not usually physically fatigued when they go to bed at night, because they are quite sedentary during the day. They are not as active as before, and therefore are not as tired by physical activity.

What can happen if these new patterns continue for many weeks? To begin with, you will develop an association between going to bed and *not* sleeping. This becomes the new habit because your nervous system learns that going to bed is a cue for being awake for the next few hours, instead of a cue for going to sleep. Have you ever noticed that you can be very tired and ready to sleep, but when your head hits the pillow you are suddenly wide awake? This is the result of the learning I am talking about.

Let us examine more closely just what can go wrong. There are three basic types of sleep disturbance which affect chronic-pain sufferers. The first is called *sleep-onset insomnia*, and it is characterized by the inability to fall asleep. People who used to go to bed and fall asleep in five to ten minutes before they were hurt or suffered a painful illness find themselves tossing and turning for an hour or more. This is partly because they are unable to get comfortable, and partly because they have conditioned themselves that going to bed does not mean falling asleep. Also, as I mentioned above, the fact that they have not expended as much physical energy during the day means that they are not as tired as they used to be at night.

The second type of sleep disturbance is that of *frequent awakening* during the night. Most people report that if they happen to turn the wrong way, the pain wakes them up. Then they have a terrible time falling back asleep. Sometimes the pain does not actually wake them up, but it still causes restless sleep, just like the patients studied by Dr. Muldofsky.

For those chronic-pain sufferers who were injured in an accident, there is a second awakening problem. They often have terrible nightmares about their accidents. These bad dreams not only wake them, but they create a lingering anxiety which prevents them from falling back to sleep. Frequent awakening is likely related to the Stage Three sleep disruption that Dr. Muldofsky observed.

The third sleep dysfunction is *early awakening*. Many people with chronic pain go to bed at a decent hour, but wake up at 3 or 4 A.M., before they've had sufficient sleep. However, sleep at this time of the morning eludes them. Sometimes this is a sign of depression, which, of course, may be associated with chronic-pain syndrome. They may toss and turn in bed in discomfort, or they might wander the house in search of some sort of relief. They may or may not eventually fall asleep, but their healthy sleep patterns have been disrupted. Moreover, the day has started off badly, and the stress of not being able to get a normal night's sleep sets them up for a miserable, painful day.

Breaking the Sleep-Pain Link

Normal sleeping patterns are long-standing habits. Those of you who suffer from chronic pain have unlearned your normal habits and have learned new, deleterious sleep patterns which contribute to your pain problem. These unhealthy sleep patterns must be changed to help you control the chronic-pain condition. The habits have to be re-programmed, and the good news is that it is within your power!

I have found that a person with chronic-pain problems who is unable to sleep properly can be trained to redevelop his former, healthy sleep patterns. We have an eight-point program, with which we have had great success. After I set out the program, I will give you an example of just how effective it can be.

1. The first step is to establish a new structure for your sleeping patterns. My experience has been that the simplest way to do this is to establish a new wake-up time in the morning, as opposed to setting a new time for going to sleep. This is because you can use an alarm clock in the morning, but you cannot guarantee the time that you will actually go to sleep.

I recommend that the new wake-up time approximate the wake-up time that you were accustomed to prior to the onset of your pain problem. After all, it is easier to re-establish an old pattern than to introduce an entirely new one.

I realize that the first few mornings of your new wake-up time will be particularly difficult, especially if you have become accustomed to rising late. But it is crucial that you adhere faithfully to this new schedule in order to defeat your sleep problem.

2. The second step in establishing a new sleep habit is to wait until you are sleepy before going to bed. Since you are now getting up at a fixed time each morning, your body will tell you when it is time for bed, depending upon its own needs.

At first, if you've been used to going to bed late, you will still have the habit of being sleepy at the later time. It will take a few days for your body to re-adjust to your new wake-up time and, naturally, you are going to be tired for these few days. After this time, I have found that the new pattern asserts itself and you will once again establish a time at which your body tells you it is time to go to sleep.

3. The most crucial step is to stop "trying" to fall asleep. You cannot force yourself to fall asleep; it is stressful and self-defeating to even try. Instead, you are now going to re-condition your sleep habit. I'll explain how to do that by way of an example.

Suppose that, for the last few months, you have been going to bed at 11 P.M. but tossing and turning until 2 A.M. when you finally fall asleep. As a consequence, you wake up in the morning feeling exhausted and irritable. You have become increasingly frustrated, uncomfortable, and angry with the situation. Before your pain problem, you used to go to bed at 11 P.M. and be asleep within twenty or thirty minutes.

What's the solution? First of all, you've already established a new waking time of 7 A.M. And now you are going to follow step two and go to bed when you feel sleepy. That may happen at eleven, or later. But instead of lying there anxiously trying to fall asleep, we want you to try a different approach. You know from the past few months' experience that you will not be asleep in a half hour. So, tell yourself, "I'm simply going to lie here for half an hour and then get up if I'm still awake." After the thirty minutes, you will get up and leave the bedroom.

The first difference you will notice about this approach is that you are not lying there fuming about not being able to sleep. You have made a conscious decision to simply lie there for the half hour. There is no need for anger because you are not "trying" to fall asleep. Of course, if you happened to fall asleep during this time, so much the better.

After you have left the bedroom you should then go to another part of your residence and do something soothing, like playing solitaire, doing a crossword puzzle, or reading something light, until you feel sleepy again. Just avoid doing anything stimulating, because it may override your sleepiness. Continue doing the activity until you feel that you are ready to go asleep again. Then return to bed. Again, check the time and inform yourself that if you are not asleep in thirty minutes, you will get up again and return to your activity.

You repeat this process until you fall asleep, which will probably be about 2 or 3 A.M. — the time you have been regularly dozing off since your chronic-pain condition began. Follow the same routine the next night.

It will take a few days, but eventually you will begin falling asleep at your new sleep time (which may or may not be at 11 P.M.). Keep up the same process until you are regularly falling asleep within the thirty-minute time frame. What you have done is retrain your body and nervous system to associate going to bed with sleep, not with the onset of sleeplessness and anxiety.

4. If you wake up at any time during the night and cannot fall asleep again within thirty minutes, resume the process described in step three.

5. Going to bed should not be associated with any activity other than sleep, *unless* that activity actually helps you relax. For example, if you find reading or watching television relaxing and conducive to dozing, it is acceptable. (Incidentally, some people find sexual activity relaxing, others stimulating — Vive la différence!) We want you to associate your bedroom primarily with going to sleep.

6. I recommend that you do not nap during the day. People who have lengthy convalescent periods after a serious injury or illness are often at home all day and have a tendency to take naps. Whether they do this primarily to kill time or to relieve discomfort of some sort is immaterial. What matters is that you are disrupting your normal sleep patterns, making it

more difficult for you to achieve a proper night's rest.

7. Start a regular exercise and activity program as I described in Chapter 7. However, do not exercise in the last two to three hours before going to bed. Physical exercise has a tendency to invigorate a person to the point where it may take a few hours to calm down enough to fall asleep.

8. Relaxation techniques can help you fall asleep under the right circumstances. First of all, you have to be well practiced at the technique and you need to follow the first seven rules I have laid out. Do not try too hard, because an overly conscious attempt to relax can have the opposite effect, just as trying hard to fall asleep can keep you awake.

My clinical experience has been that, if our patients carefully follow the above rules, they return to normal sleep within three to four days. Our success rate is about ninety per cent, although the patients often go through a tough time during the retraining period. If this happens to you, don't become immediately discouraged and give up on your program. The chronic-pain/sleep-disturbance link is not always broken easily. However, three or four days of less sleep and more fatigue is a small price to pay for long-term renewal of normal sleep habits.

I caution you not to think that you have totally defeated the problem after your first good night's sleep. Old habits are hard to break, and you may have the same trouble falling asleep on the fifth or sixth night. If that happens, you have to once again repeat the retraining process.

A Bed of Roses

A lot of people with chronic pain blame their inability to sleep at night on their bedding, and there is no doubt that it is difficult to feel comfortable when you are lying on what feels like a bed of thorns. So, it is important for you to have a proper mattress and pillows.

There are no hard-and-fast rules when it comes to choosing a mattress, because no two bodies are alike. For example, some people swear by waterbeds; others swear at them. There are those who are comfortable only when lying on rock-hard mattresses, but many can sleep comfortably only on soft ones. You will simply have to experiment until you find the right one for you. Just remember to give each mattress a few days' trial; it is not possible to determine after one night whether or not one is right or wrong for you.

Propping yourself up on a mountain of pillows will not automatically make you feel better. In fact, if you have a neck or back problem, pillows may actually aggravate your condition. Some people with a low-back problem feel better if they sleep with a small pillow between their knees (if they lie on their side). Others might find relief if they lie on their backs with pillows under their knees, which are raised and bent. Once again, you must experiment to see if and how the placement of pillows can help you to sleep better.

The same advice applies to chronic neck pain. Many people have experienced relief by using special "orthopedic" pillows, which are contoured to conform to the shape of a normal cervical-spinal column. They appear to be useful for osteoarthritic conditions in the neck, which are caused by normal wear-and-tear of the joints in that area. When people wake up in the morning with a lot more pain than they had when they went to bed, it is a signal that the pillows on which they rest are not providing their necks with proper positioning while they sleep.

The final advice I have for people in search of a comfortable bed and pillows is to *try only one new thing at a time*. You may never know, otherwise, exactly what helped or irritated you. And you can waste a lot of time and money trying to find out. So, try a new pillow first if you have a neck problem. Try it for several consecutive nights. If you have a back problem, try positioning some pillows differently, as I described above. If that does not provide relief, try a new mattress. It will not take that long before you discover what really helps you sleep better.

An easy and seemingly innocuous way of overcoming an inability to sleep is a sleeping pill. There are countless commercials on television for "safe" drugs to induce sleep. The shelves of your local pharmacy are full of prescription and over-the-counter drugs. There is very little wrong with these medications if they are used sparingly for only for a day or two when stress interferes with normal sleep. But used over the long run, these "harmless" pills can become addictive crutches. As I will explain in Chapter 15, no drugs are perfectly safe in the long run, and they only prolong the time before you must take steps to deal with the pain problem for good.

Another chemical fix is alcohol. How often have you taken a little "shot" of something to help you relax and fall asleep at night? That shot may eventually become a larger glassful, and you may end up with a different problem. Furthermore, alcohol, like caffeine, tends to disturb normal sleeping patterns if consumed in sufficient quantities. (The amount varies with each individual.) Have you ever had a fairly large amount of alcohol to drink in the evening, fallen asleep quickly, only to find yourself wide awake in the middle of the night and unable to get back to sleep? I can assure you that my system works better than alcohol or sleeping pills. Let me end this chapter with one more example.

I once treated a woman who had been unable to fall asleep without sleeping pills for *five* years and she desperately wanted to break her dependency. I convinced her to try the eight-step retraining approach, but I stressed to her the need to consult her doctor first before totally stopping the sleeping pills. She did exactly as I told her, except that she immediately threw away her sleeping pills without consulting her doctor.

It took her three nights to train herself to sleep normally. She called to tell me that she had slept peacefully for the whole night and awakened refreshed, without pills, for the first time in five years. I cautioned her that her old sleeping habits might return before they disappeared for good, and advised her to call me if she had any problem. A few weeks later she called to say that she had needed to repeat the process once again, but the problem now seemed to be under control.

You too can achieve this kind of outcome if you stick to it and take control of your own sleeping patterns.

CHAPTER

15

Medication: Bittersweet Pills

~~~~~~~~~~

One of the best things about analgesics — painkilling medications — is that, when administered properly, they work. One of the *worst* things about them is that they work so well. Their popularity leads chronic-pain patients to see them as long-term solutions when they are not, and precludes the patients' looking to other pain-control strategies.

Painkilling medications are both blessings and curses in disguise. As with all drugs, the problem with them is that there is a strong potential for side effects as well as abuse. Analgesics may even help perpetuate a chronic-pain condition, as we shall see shortly. It is important to offer chronic-pain sufferers strategies for pain control that effectively remove the need for long-term medications.

Analgesics and Chronic Pain

There is no doubt that analgesics play a crucial role in the management of acute pain, because they relieve discomfort quickly and effectively. Furthermore, once the cause of the acute pain has been removed, the need for the drugs disappears and there is no concern over their potential side effects.

Unfortunately, such is not the case with chronic pain. The chronic-pain sufferer may take medication for months or years, thereby risking some serious problems — such as tolerance or addiction.

Tolerance means that your nervous system becomes accustomed to the action of the drug, and therefore less sensitive to it. It requires more and more of the drug to provide the same painkilling relief. Tolerance is related to dependency, in that your body becomes so used to having the drug in the bloodstream that it starts to need it. This is also the basis of addiction.

Anti-inflammatories, anti-depressants, muscle relaxants, and tranquilizers may often help reduce pain, but the extent of their use pales in comparison to that of analgesics, partly because so many painkillers are available over the counter and some are undeniably effective. However, any analgesic can be harmful if used too frequently or for too long a period of time. Using them in this way should be monitored by physicians who have fully explained their possible long-term effects.

Most analgesics are relatively safe if used sparingly. The major ingredient is usually ASA or acetaminophen which are well known painkillers. A few are available that contain codeine, which is a more powerful painkilling substance. Codeine has more side effects, the most serious being addiction.

Some analgesics, like Talwin and Demerol, are derived from morphine, and are therefore stronger than other drugs. They are available by prescription only, and while certainly effective against pain can produce a powerful addiction. It is thought that these chemicals take the place of endorphins, which is why they are so powerful. For this reason, there is a chance over the long run that they alter the normal functioning of your pain system. Isn't it better to retain control over your pain system rather than having to rely upon artificial supports?

When I first began treating chronic-pain sufferers I was amazed that they regularly took painkillers even though they often admitted that the drugs were really not very effective. When I questioned their continued use of something that gave little relief, they pointed to the fact that the doctor was still prescribing them, and they hadn't questioned the prescription renewal. Others told me they were just plain desperate. They did not know what else to do! These people would have been happy to dump all their pills down the toilet, but they did not know how to cope afterward. They couldn't part with their "crutches", even though the drugs could not keep them pain free.

I have seen a few patients who had taken drugs for many years to kill pain, and who had developed an addiction. Some of them had reached the point where their addiction problems superseded their chronic-pain behavior patterns. But they are the exceptions rather than the norm. I find that most people take painkilling drugs even though they don't want to, simply because they don't know what else to do.

Chronic-pain victims often have a whole medicine cabinet full of drugs. Some are over-the-counter medications recommended to them by friends and relatives. A few have been prescribed for other people who are eager to help. Others, of course, have been prescribed by their doctors.

In almost every case, they take the drug "as needed." That is, they wait until the pain has built up to the point that they begin to feel uncomfortable or feel they soon will become so. When I ask why they do this, they tell me that they really don't like taking the drugs, so they hold off as long as they comfortably can. In their minds, taking the drug is an admission of their failure to manage the pain. As we shall soon learn, taking analgesics on an "as needed" basis is a bad strategy for chronic pain.

Some people who do not want to continue taking painkillers actually throw out all their drugs and go "cold turkey."

This may work occasionally, but the person can have side effects from the sudden withdrawal of drugs that have been in his or her system for a long time. There can also be a "boomerang effect" — the pain hits with a vengeance, and the person is then forced to return to the medications to obtain relief. This is like throwing away your crutches right after breaking a leg and putting all your weight on your injured limb before it heals; it will flare up from the sudden demands you place on it.

This does not mean that once you have been taking pain-killers for a long time, you will never be able to live without them. However, I strongly recommend that withdrawal from the medication be gradual, and that the drugs be replaced by other pain-relieving methods — such as relaxation therapies.

The object of this chapter, however, is not to list a whole range of drugs and their potentially harmful effects. For one thing, the list changes rapidly, and also it would take an entire book to do justice to the subject. What I want to focus on is the fact that chronic-pain management need not revolve around potentially harmful drugs. There *is* an alternative.

Do Not Take as Needed

The first problem with taking painkillers "as needed" is that most people wait and medicate themselves only when their discomfort levels are at their highest. It then takes a while for the drugs to enter the bloodstream and affect the pain system. During that half hour or so, the person may become quite anxious and impatient. On the other hand, he may lie down immediately, and if the pain subsides it may be due to his resting, not to medication. Therefore, it is often difficult to ascertain the actual effect of the drug.

In addition, most chronic-pain sufferers hate being "pill-poppers" and they become angry with themselves when they are finally forced by pain to take medication. They are like the people who cannot fall asleep; their frustration makes them more angry and anxious, which in turn feeds their pain systems and causes them more discomfort.

Finally, since it takes some time for the drug to enter the bloodstream, it cannot work in a preventative way to take the edge off the worst peaks of pain.

However, my main concern with "as needed" schedules is that the person is actually reinforcing behaviors he or she does not want. How does this happen? If you look at the graph (Figure 12), you will more easily understand this point.

As you can see, there are peaks and valleys in this person's pain levels during the day. This pain sufferer waits until the pain is reaching its peak before taking his or her painkiller. In this case taking the drug is quickly followed by a reduction in discomfort and perhaps some pleasant side effects from the drug, such as a mild euphoria. Therefore, each pain peak is followed by a pleasant drug state as well as a rapid improvement in the amount of pain. Since we know that conditioning is based upon the repeated association of events in time, you can see that there is a continued linking of high pain with drug intake and less pain. This can result in reinforcing the drug-taking behavior and the pain behavior that accompa-

FIGURE 12   *Pain, and Medication "As Needed"*

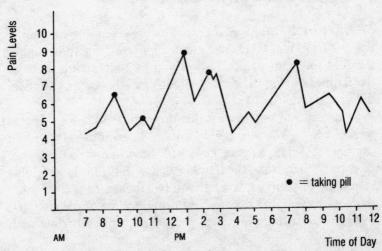

nies the pain peaks. These are behaviors that you do not want.

A few hours after medication has been taken, the pain has returned to an intolerable level, so the sufferer takes another analgesic. The cycle may continue for the entire day and for a period of many years, becoming an ingrained pattern.

There are three steps you can take to solve this problem and to help you to gradually stop taking analgesics. This procedure will place you in better control of your pain without the need for the drugs.

Step 1: Monitoring To begin with, you should monitor your medications and pain as I described in Chapter 6. After you have done this for at least one week, count up the number of pills you have taken each day over the week. Let us say you took five pills on day one, four on day two, seven on the third day, two on the fourth, three on day five, nine on the sixth day, and five on the seventh. In one week you took thirty-five pills, an average of five per day. Therefore, your baseline is five pills per day.

When you review your monitoring, check to see if the pills had a significant effect on your pain. Did your pain levels drop a couple of levels each time you took a pill? If not, this is all the more reason to get rid of them.

Step 2: Fixed Time Schedule Now we are going to change the cue for when you take those analgesics. Instead of taking them at the pain peaks, I want you to start taking them at fixed times during the day. Now the clock becomes your cue, not your pain.

I suggest that you discuss this procedure with your doctor to see if he or she is agreeable. If so, I recommend that you use your baseline as your gauge for how many you take per day. In our example, the baseline is five pills per day and this should be the starting level. If you feel that there will be some days when you will be sorely tempted to take more than the five, I suggest that you start off the fixed time schedule with six per day. *The most important principle here is that you take the drugs according to the clock and not according to your pain.*

At this point you might protest, "But that means that some days I'll take five pills even though I only need two. Isn't that bad for me?" The answer is that this is only your starting level and the purpose is to wean you eventually off this unnecessary medication entirely. But we are doing it the smart, systematic way, the way that works best for most chronic-pain sufferers.

I want you to continue taking the five (or six) pills a day, every day, at the beginning. How do you establish the best times to actually take the pills? Again, get permission from your doctor about this, but I suggest that you divide them evenly throughout the day as is shown in Figure 13. This graph is from the same person as Figure 12. Notice how the analgesics are now taken at 7 A.M., 11 A.M., 3 P.M., 7 P.M., and 11 P.M.. Also notice how the pain peaks have been smoothed out. This person now has the medication in his bloodstream when he most needs it (*before* the pain builds up) and it is working as a pain preventative. Secondly, taking the pill is no longer a

FIGURE 13   *Pain, and Medication "To Schedule"*

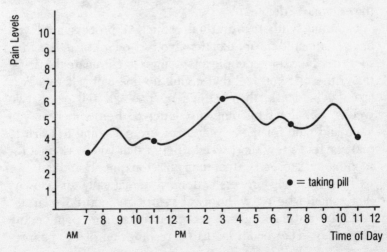

cause for guilt or indecision; he is following a new schedule to wean him from the drugs.

Now that you are on a regulated, fixed dosage of the analgesic you can maintain this for several weeks, until the situation has stabilized and you can take the next step. Remember to take the pills regularly, regardless of how you feel. If you hit a tough spot, use relaxation or imagery or anxiolytic exercise for pain control, but do not take the next pill until the designated time. You will find that it gets easier as time goes on.

Step 3: Reducing the Dosage The next step is to reduce the number of pills you are taking. Again, this is done slowly and gradually using the principles of shaping instead of using pain as the cue.

Let us go back to our example. The baseline is five pills a day, so the first step is to drop to four and a half pills a day by cutting one of them in half. (If you are using capsules, consult your doctor who might be able to offer alternative medications.) After one week at this new level you might reduce the dosage to four pills a day. Note that this second reduction does not have to be at the same time as the one that you cut in half the first time. You can pick any of the designated times as the next one to delete.

Continue with this gradual reduction process until you have eliminated the medication. No two people are the same, so it may take some people a lot longer to eliminate the drugs than others. If you feel that giving up one-half pill a week is too much to ask, then reduce by one-half pill every two weeks, but don't become discouraged. Remember, if you have had pain for many years, you are not going to learn to manage it in a few short weeks. Better that you work on it for months and succeed, rather than push too quickly and fail.

If the weaning process is done systematically and slowly, there should be no withdrawal symptoms and no relapses. You must not backtrack if you experience more pain on any given day. That could lead to a resumption of the pain-reinforcement link. Instead, use your newly acquired pain-control techniques. Our experience has been that these techniques work quite well, in fact better than the medications upon which you previously relied.

I must admit that not everyone is able to totally give up painkilling medication. However, those that cannot are at least able to substantially reduce their intake — an important step, considering the potential long-term problems that may be associated with analgesics. If you are unable to eliminate painkillers altogether, then remember to stick to the fixed-time schedule without fail, as this is your best chance of continuing to manage your pain problem in the future. Of course the ideal is to totally eliminate drug-taking to control pain.

The Other Pills in Your Medicine Cabinet

Although I have concentrated on analgesics in this chapter, I should point out that other medications are also popular for the management of chronic pain. These drugs include anti-inflammatories, muscle-relaxants, tranquilizers and anti-depressants. In some cases — for instance, systemic disorders such as rheumatoid arthritis — these drugs are effective treatments and I certainly support their continued use. Each of these drugs is potentially beneficial, but its benefits must be weighed against the possible harm in each case.

As you would expect, anti-inflammatory medications reduce inflammation in joints and in soft tissue regardless of the cause of the inflammation. Anti-inflammatories also have analgesic properties independent of their anti-inflammatory action. You can develop a tolerance to the action of these drugs, and many people complain of unpleasant gastrointestinal side effects caused by anti-inflammatories. In view of the proliferation of anti-inflammatories in the last few years, most people who require them should be able to find one that is fairly safe for them. The selection has to be worked out between you and your doctor.

Other drugs that may be prescribed for pain control are muscle-relaxants and tranquilizers, which belong to the same family of medications. They can be effective in the short run, because they help to relax tense muscles and they aid those who have anxiety or trouble falling asleep. But they have many drawbacks if they are taken for long periods of time. Muscle-relaxants are not a replacement for learning how to

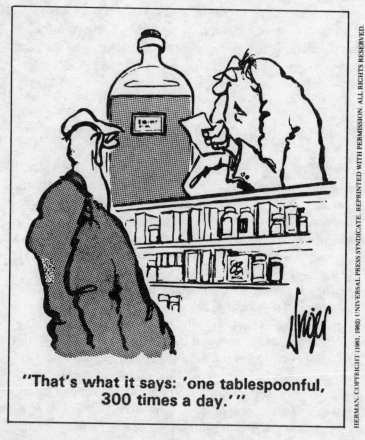

"That's what it says: 'one tablespoonful, 300 times a day.'"

The danger of over-medication.

relax, because they do not teach you how to manage the problem for yourself. You also develop a tolerance to their action so that you need more and more for the same effect. In addition, you can become quickly dependent on these drugs, and withdrawal from them can produce serious emotional problems. Once again, a patient must discuss these drugs thoroughly with a medical professional so as to understand the benefits and drawbacks of their long-term use.

I have already discussed antidepressants with regard to their neurochemical action. Compared to tranquilizers, there appear to be fewer side effects with this class of drugs. Dependency is rare although rapid withdrawal can trigger a "boomerang effect" (i.e. a recurrence). However, the greatest difficulty that I have seen with these drugs is the inability of people to endure the short-term side effects, such as dry mouth, tremors, etc. For some people these side effects are too unpleasant to justify the use of the drug.

In order to eliminate the use of all these drugs, you must learn alternative approaches to pain control. The scheduling and reduction process that I described in this chapter for analgesics applies equally well to these other medications. Be sure that you discuss the steps with your physician, and remember to take it gradually. It takes a while to learn these new techniques — to replace old habits with new ones, but at least for the first time in many months you will be in control.

CHAPTER 16

The Alphabet of Treatments

All too many chronic-pain patients take a scatter-gun approach in dealing with their problem. Many of the patients I see have run the gamut of treatments for their chronic pain, from acupuncture to Zen Buddhism. Their hope is that, by trying everything, a cure will suddenly take place. That may happen in a rare case, but usually these people end up wasting a lot of time and money, and suffering prolonged and unnecessary physical and emotional distress. That's usually what has happened by the time they show up at my clinic.

Despite these failures, I know that many chronic-pain patients attempt alternative therapies for many reasons. Each therapy has its success stories, and it is always heartening to know that some people can be helped by these means. If you are going to try one of them, I suggest that you become an educated consumer. I want you to know what is available out there and how to evaluate it from a cognitive-behavioral perspective. After listing the criteria for judging treatments, we will briefly examine some of the alternatives available.

Buyer Beware

1. Most of the treatments lack the *multi-dimensional* approach of the program I have laid out in this book. This is because the majority of them are better suited to acute rather than to chronic problems. Acute pain is normally treatable by attacking the specific cause of the discomfort, such as an inflamed joint, a pulled ligament, etc. As you now know, chronic-pain conditions are much more complex than this, and consequently they require a multi-dimensional approach, which takes into account *all* the factors affecting the pain system.

Ironically, each individual therapy is probably solving its own piece of the puzzle. But since other factors are also feeding into the pain system, the good you do in this one small area is outweighed by the others. Take massage as an example.

Massage can be useful in reducing muscle tension, but the effects are very short-lived. This shouldn't surprise us since there are several triggers for muscle tension, including poor posture, stress, anxiety, and muscular habits. These triggers are always present since, in essence, the patient carries them with him or her. Is it any wonder that the muscle tension and pain return with a vengeance within a few hours after massage? Only if therapies to resolve these other triggers are used in the correct combination can the muscles be *kept* relaxed long after the masseur is finished.

2. The second problem with many treatments for chronic pain is that they tend to be *passive*. If you are receiving treatment such as medication, massage, manipulation, etc. in which you are the *recipient* of therapy prescribed by and carried out by others, you are dealing with your pain problem passively.

Clinical experience and research indicates that most chronic-pain victims require an *active* approach to therapy — for example, a program of exercises and other cognitive-behavioral strategies. They have to learn how to actively manage their pain problems before they can experience long-term relief. With passive treatments, you are not learning anything positive about your situation; in fact you may be blocking your chances for improvement, because you are not developing strategies to manage your pain problem.

3.   Treatments cannot simply go on forever, as much as some therapists would like them to. There is an *adequate therapeutic trial* for each type of treatment, and you should ask the practitioner of any therapy what that time frame is before you begin treatment. It is most likely to be two or three months, not a matter of a year or two. All too often patients continue with a therapy long after it has proven to be clinically ineffective for them. You should be able to rely on the health-care provider to know the proper time frame and to tell you about it, but this is not always the case.

Once you have given a therapy an adequate therapeutic trial and it is not working, you should discontinue it. You must understand that the longer an ineffective therapy goes on, the more deeply the pain pattern becomes ingrained in your nervous system. This is not so much the fault of the technique you have been using, as it is owing to the fact that time is continuing to pass without you getting the help you need to get better. For example, one of the concerns that cancer specialists have about experimental treatments like laetrile is that, for however long the patient is using the drug, he or she is not getting the benefit of chemotherapy or radiation or other treatments which have been proven to be effective.

4.   The next problem is that *short-term relief* does not add up to long-term cure. One of the worst difficulties with passive therapies is that they often provide dramatic pain reduction for a few hours, or as long as a day, and then the pain returns at its old level. After this pattern repeats over a period of weeks, the patient naturally becomes discouraged. If this keeps happening, it is a sign that the therapy is either not addressing the underlying cause for the pain or that the solu-

tion needs to be multi-dimensional. Unfortunately, it is difficult for patients in this position to break away from a therapy like this because they welcome even the little pain relief they are getting and they cherish the frail hope that they will improve over the long term.

5.   Techniques which provide short-term relief often foster an unhealthy *dependence* on the therapist and therapeutic devices. All too often I have seen people who have been receiving chiropractic treatment, or massage, ultrasound, acupuncture, TENS (Transcutaneous Electrical Nerve Stimulation), etc. for years, and their overall level of pain is no better than it was when they started. But they cling to it out of desperation, and develop an almost child-like dependency on the therapist. Imagine how much better off they would be had they invested all that time and energy in taking an active approach and learning their own pain-control skills?

6.   Because the study of pain is in its infancy, it is wise to take any *startling claims* that are made by new therapies with a grain of salt. Just because one may claim to have found a "trigger point", or a way of manipulating the spine to temporarily relieve pain, does not mean that the problem has been permanently solved. Remember that there is usually more than one reason for chronic pain, so *all* these reasons must be addressed by combining a whole range of therapeutic techniques.

7.   Then there is the *placebo effect*. Research has shown that about thirty per cent of all people will respond favorably to *any* treatment, because of the placebo effect. If they *believe* they are getting therapy that works, they will experience short-term relief. If their problems are transitory, they will be cured without knowing if the treatment was effective, over and above the placebo effect. But if they suffer from long-term pain, they will probably learn soon enough that their problems are not yet solved, because the chronic discomfort will return.

As I mentioned previously, the placebo effect is caused by the release of endorphins. Placebos are non-invasive and very safe, as long as they do not preclude more appropriate treatments. At a minimum, you should find out if the therapy you are undergoing has been compared to a placebo treatment in a controlled study.

8.   If you get a backache for the first time, you should be aware that the vast majority of back-pain problems disappears completely within six months, *whether or not you receive any treatment*. This automatic recovery process is known as *spontaneous remission*. This is a factor that you should be aware of because there is always a chance that you incorrectly attribute your recovery to a treatment when in fact you recovered spontaneously.

However, as I have mentioned before, the spontaneous remission rate for chronic pain of two years' duration or longer is approximately fifteen per cent. Therefore, if you are in this position, the chance that your recovery is spontaneous is very unlikely.

9.   Your *responsibility* and the responsibility of the therapist should be clear to you. You must communicate extensively with the people treating you to understand your own role in the treatment, because failure to do so will jeopardize your attempts to obtain relief. The therapist must take the time to explain the important elements of the therapy and to advise you what to expect.

You also need to know what is expected of you and what you can do to assist the therapeutic process. It is important to carefully follow the instructions laid out for you by your therapist. All too often patients fail to take medications as prescribed, or they ignore exercise programs they are told to follow. They believe that only a simple, quick fix can cure them, and they have no patience with multi-dimensional approaches that take time to work effectively. Unfortunately, if the treatment fails, they have no one to blame but themselves.

The Unkindest Cut

People who suffer from severe chronic pain often choose a surgical solution in an attempt to find relief, even though they may have been warned that success is not guaranteed. Their rationale is "I can't get any worse." Unfortunately, some do, although in other cases the positive effects of surgery are dramatic.

I caution all those contemplating an operation to get at least two opinions from qualified medical experts. Despite the skills of surgeons today, no operation is without an element of risk. Moreover, there is the problem of scar tissue, which forms naturally at the site of an incision and can create more pain than existed before the operation. I do not want to scare people away from surgery, particularly when it is essential rather than elective. However, you must be fully aware of the potential complications of any invasive procedure.

Some people have nerves severed or deadened by various means in an attempt to stop pain. But these procedures have mixed success rates and, even worse, can have horrible side effects. I remember one man who told me that he had gone through a rhizotomy to deaden some pain in his cheekbone. A rhizotomy involves the burning out of nerves by passing a strong electrical current through them. Although the cheekbone pain was cured, the patient was left with excruciating constant pain on his forehead owing to the destruction of the nerve.

Needlework

Surgery is not the only invasive procedure applied to pain control. There are all kinds of needles used by health-care professionals to perform a variety of treatments.

The needlework best known in medical clinics today is *acupuncture*, which I will explain only very briefly. The ancient theory was that acupuncture somehow balanced the yin and yang in a person's body. This explanation proved too unscientific for occidental minds, which may account for the fact that it was only recently accepted by Western medical professionals to any degree. Its acceptance owes much to the gate-control theory and to the apparent fact that acupuncture activates the release of endorphins.

Unfortunately, there are many people who experience either no relief after acupuncture treatments, or only transitory relief. Chronic-pain sufferers who do experience short-term relief may become regular acupuncture patients. Thus, they become passive patients who fail to play an active role in their own treatment program. As I mentioned above, this situation is not conducive to effective chronic-pain management.

Notwithstanding this, I believe that acupuncture is worth trying. There have been some dramatic success stories of the complete disappearance of a pain condition. Some acupuncturists pass an electric current through the needles, which makes the procedure somewhat like an invasive form of TENS (see below). Other experts twirl the needles once they have been placed in position in the skin, and there are those who treat the needles with special herbal medications. You may wish to seek out different practitioners if one method does not work for you.

For those who are frightened by needles, there is now *laser acupuncture*, which apparently works equally well or poorly depending upon your point of view. Laser acupuncture has the advantage over traditional acupuncture of not using needles to pierce the skin. This eliminates the chance of infection. Regardless of the technique, I recommend that you use only a registered practitioner.

Some doctors treat a pain condition by injecting *local anesthetics* into a painful area. This treatment is often tried on people with severe low-back pain. The anesthetic can work wonders for certain neurological or musculoskeletal disorders, at least in the short run. But the procedure often fails to provide long-term relief.

I have seen people who have become regular recipients of these anesthetic injections. One might say that the patient has actually become "injection dependent". If your experience with these injections has been one of short-term relief only, and you have been going for many months without an overall reduction in pain, I would advise you to give it up. You are hindering your goal to achieve an effective pain-management program, which includes your *active* participation.

Another type of injection that is used in painful conditions is *cortisone*. However, one has to be extremely cautious about the liberal use of cortisone shots, because in the long run they may hasten the destruction of the joints into which they are frequently injected. Also, steroids in general carry with them many potentially deleterious side effects.

Relief in a Bottle

In the last chapter I discussed the use of drugs to control chronic pain, so I will not dwell on the benefits and problems they provide here. The pain system is also affected by alcohol, which can, of course, be addictive. It can also cause depression and a variety of physical problems if abused. Finally, alcohol is not a very good analgesic anyway, as people will discover if they monitor their pain over a period of time. There are far more effective ways of handling a pain problem than drowning it in booze.

The Medium Is the Masseur

There are so many ways of therapeutically manipulating or massaging the body that it would take an entire book to describe them all adequately. Some people find chiropractors helpful in this department, others rely on shiatsu therapists, and so on. If this form of treatment makes you feel good, then by all means go for it. This may sound like a broken record, but the big problem with massage/manipulation is that many people are helped only in the short run.

"I threw my back out last year and I went to the chiropractor [or masseur] for a month or so, and I was fine for almost a year. Then my back went out again, and I returned to him for a few more sessions. He fixed me up for a few weeks, but I had to see him again recently for another treatment. He's great . . . helps me whenever the old back acts up".

Does that monologue sound familiar? If this person realized that there was much more that could be done to prevent and control these pain episodes, I wonder if he would see his treatment regimen as a solution or as part of the problem? I take the latter view!

There is no doubt that manipulators/masseurs help many people who are in pain. In fact, we often utilize such treatments for certain types of pain problems, as long as they are carried out in conjunction with a comprehensive pain-management program. When they are utilized exclusively, however, they can end up simply being a "Band-Aid" approach.

I have been impressed with the effectiveness of spinal manipulations performed by chiropractors. Also, some of them have taken off their blinkers and have begun to combine their treatments with exercise and other regimens. Still, I am told by my medical colleagues that chiropractic theory rests on shaky ground and this might be an instance where the treatment works — but not for the reasons the chiropractors believe.

My biggest complaint about chiropractic treatment has to do with the failure to establish the duration of an adequate therapeutic trial. All too often I see people who have been going to a chiropractor for many months, or even years, and who are receiving minimal short-term relief, but who are really no better than when they started.

What I said about chiropractors also applies to massage therapists. If their treatment is combined with a comprehensive program, it can be quite beneficial, particularly for those people who suffer a great deal from muscle tension. Many people are helped by more gentle massages; others benefit more from rigorous techniques, such as Swedish massage, shiatsu, or rolfing. These methods seem to be based on counter-irritation theories — i.e. you irritate a painful area even further to stimulate the closure of the "gate", thereby preventing pain messages from reaching the brain.

Physiotherapy

Physiotherapy encompasses a wide variety of treatment techniques ranging from hot packs to cold packs, passive to active treatments, and rest to exercise. They include manipulation, massage, joint-mobilization, exercise, traction, ultrasound, TENS, postural training, gait-training, and much more. A physiotherapist's repertoire is most impressive.

As you can see, physiotherapy can take both active or passive forms. The active components can be a vital part of an overall chronic-pain treatment program. Our patients are regularly seen and advised by physiotherapists, so that they receive whatever treatments are necessary and they learn to perform their exercises properly.

I have no intention here of setting out a comprehensive exercise program because every patient is different. Exercise programs must be individualized because doing the wrong exercise can be worse than doing none at all, while doing the right ones the right way can produce dramatic results.

If you have a particular back problem, you will require one set of exercises and treatments. If your neck is the problem, you will need another program entirely, because different muscles, bones, and joints are involved. Exercise programs are essential, because they help patients break their passive habits. It will be much easier to break those habits if the exercises are the correct ones, done properly.

If you decide to undertake a specific exercise program that you have found in a book, please be careful. If you do not have an expert watching you do the exercises, you may perform them incorrectly. You run the risk of injury at worst, and wasting your time at best. I strongly urge you to seek professional advice before undertaking any complicated exercise program on your own, particularly since the diagrams and explanations in a book are often more confusing than enlightening.

Getting on One's Nerves

There are two basic ways of stimulating nerves in an attempt to "short-circuit" pain, one invasive and the other non-invasive. The most common, and non-invasive, technique is called *Transcutaneous Electrical Nerve Stimulation (TENS)*. Electrodes (either two or four) are taped to the skin at or near the pain site and, when actuated, they stimulate the nerve endings just under the skin.

The effectiveness of TENS seems to be limited to the early days of its usage. People tend to develop a tolerance to TENS after a few weeks or months and its value gradually diminishes. Patients may keep using it, because they have become dependent on the apparatus, particularly since they know of no alternatives.

In some instances we use TENS as a temporary adjunct to cognitive-behavioral therapy. The only notable side effect to the use of TENS equipment is the occasional skin irritation from the sticky tape with which it is attached to the skin.

Percutaneous Electrical Nerve Stimulation involves the implantation of an electrical stimulator near the spinal cord. The device is controlled by the patient with an external transmitter. The patient will usually activate the stimulator for about ten minutes each hour to provide constant pain relief, although the treatment regimen will vary depending on the person's condition.

This treatment is designed to benefit those with otherwise intractable pain. As you can imagine, this is a "last resort". The implantation of the electrical device is an invasive procedure; in fact it usually requires two procedures to ensure that the internal and external components are working in harmony with each other. So you would want to think twice

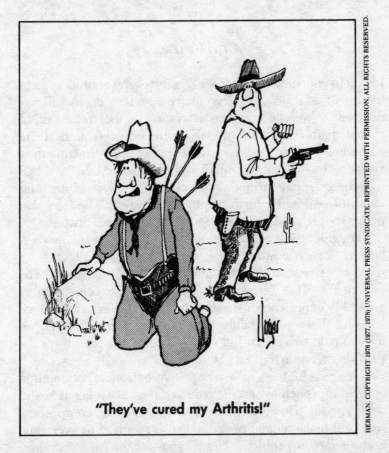

"They've cured my Arthritis!"

First use of acupuncture in North America?

about undergoing it, particularly since it works in only about fifty per cent of patients. But it is useful for pain resulting from several types of nerve damage.

If you are at the end of your pain rope and have tried most, if not all, of the above-mentioned therapies, you might be interested to learn that a few neurosurgeons are now placing similar electrical stimulators in the brain itself. They apparently have about a thirty per cent success rate over the long run.

Mind Games

I want to conclude this chapter by addressing another type of treatment — *psychiatry*. Psychiatrists and I are generally on different wavelengths when it comes to the treatment of chronic pain. They tend to look for the supposed underlying emotional reasons for chronic pain, rather than directing their attention to the pain complaints themselves. Many psychiatrists believe that chronic-pain sufferers are channelling their inner turmoil into a form of physical distress. They say that pain is the physical manifestation of the emotional distress.

They might argue that patients "need" pain to achieve certain goals, such as attracting attention, sympathy, affection, or some other reward they are otherwise unable to obtain. The patient therefore "creates" his or her pain to achieve these goals. My experience is that this is hardly the norm for chronic-pain sufferers. Certainly, attention and sympathy can reinforce pain behaviors, but they are rarely the reason for the pain's existence in the first place.

Some psychiatrists have a cognitive-behavioral orientation in their approach to chronic pain and they use relaxation and self-hypnosis. However, theirs is not usually the comprehensive pain-management program that is required to overcome a chronic-pain problem. Unless you also modify your lifestyle, your sleeping patterns, your medication intake, your pain behaviors, your cognitions, your imagery, your belief systems, and retrain your body, rebuild your stamina, and learn pacing strategies, you are not likely to totally beat chronic pain.

Psychiatrists use tranquilizers and anti-depressants liberally to control pain. That's fine if they work well and help solve the chronic-pain problem. But we now know that this approach is one-dimensional, and therefore not likely to be effective in the long run.

The bottom line here is that psychiatrists have limited success in treating chronic-pain sufferers, and I suspect that most psychiatrists would agree with me. In fact, most psychiatrists I know are reluctant to accept chronic-pain victims as patients because their success rates are so low.

How Does our Therapy Measure Up to these Principles?

Let us take a look at each principle separately:

1. Multi-dimensional: This is a strong point of cognitive-behavioral therapy. Most of the important therapies can be and are incorporated into our approach, leaving no stone unturned.

2. Passive vs. active: For the most part cognitive-behavioral therapy eschews passive therapies and emphasizes active ones. The only exceptions to this principle are those cases in which there is a need to incorporate passive therapies to meet the principle of multi-dimensional treatment.

Being an active participant in your recovery means that you regain control over your life as you gain control over your pain. Furthermore, after treatment has ended you take with you all the skills you have learned, and which you can continue to use to manage recurrences or additional problems that might occur throughout the rest of your life.

3. Adequate therapeutic trial: I advise my patients that if

cognitive-behavioral therapy does not begin to help them after two or three months, it probably will not work. It is rare for a person to be helped by this technique if no breakthrough is made during the first two months. This means that you do not have to invest unreasonable amounts of time and energy in an approach that does not work for you.

4.   Duration of relief: Some aspects of cognitive-behavioral therapy, such as relaxation and self-hypnosis, do provide only short-term relief from pain. However, repetition of these strategies has a cumulative effect and, since they are combined in a multi-dimensional approach, they interact with other strategies to produce the most effective result possible.

5.   Dependence: There is no danger of dependence in cognitive-behavioral therapy, because after all the therapist is not doing anything to you — you are doing it yourself! And if you can't depend on yourself, who can you depend on?

6.   Startling claims: Cognitive-behavioral therapy is scientifically based and does not make claims that cannot be backed up with research.

7.   Placebo effect: Like all other therapies cognitive-behavioral therapy probably has a placebo effect. But since the success rate is more than double the thirty per cent rate of the placebo effect, it is clear that there is much more than this going on.

8.   Spontaneous remission: Like any other therapy, cognitive-behavioral approaches have to demonstrate that they surpass the expected recovery level produced by spontaneous remission in order to be taken seriously. This has been verified by the scientific research in the field.

9.   Responsibility: Cognitive-behavioral therapy emphasizes the joint responsibilities of the therapist and the patient. Since the patient is an active participant in therapy, he or she is taking responsibility on a daily basis.

The fact that patients take on the responsibility for their

own care is demonstrated by the way that they continue managing their pain problems long after they have left the program. In one study we found that almost all our successful patients were doing well eighteen months following the end of treatment.

I want you to leave this chapter understanding that all the treatment techniques I describe above can provide relief for *some* chronic-pain sufferers. Unfortunately, they regularly fail to overcome chronic-pain conditions for many people, at least by themselves. What is needed is a package to treat the whole patient; you cannot separate the mind, the emotions, and the body of a person, for they are biochemically united.

CHAPTER

17

Questions

Although I have tried in this book to give as much information about chronic pain as possible, here are some questions that my patients frequently ask and that I feel may be of general interest.

1. *How can you claim to effectively treat chronic pain when experts don't completely understand how the pain system works?*

There are many disease processes that are not fully understood, yet they are often treated quite successfully. We know that aspirin helps reduce fever and inflammation in certain situations, but we aren't sure why. Certain types of drugs are very useful in treating migraine headaches, although we really don't know why.

Chronic pain is a disorder (not a disease) which responds well to therapies for reasons we do not yet understand completely. But we do know enough about the pain system at this time to affect its course in many cases. Therefore we feel comfortable with our modes of treatment. Of course, the more we learn about the pain system, the better the treatment programs will become.

2. *I am having trouble managing my pain problem even with the help of your book. However, I do not have access in my community to a "pain clinic", at least not one specializing in your approach. What can I do? What should I look for in any pain clinic?*

First of all, I don't expect that everyone reading this book will be able to obtain satisfactory relief without some sort of professional help. Secondly, if you don't know of a pain clinic in your area, you can ask your family physician or your specialist for clinic names.

Naturally, I would recommend a chronic-pain clinic that uses a cognitive-behavioral approach. However, if you cannot find one, but still wish to pursue a pain-management program, there are certain things to look for in any pain clinic. Try to find one which has several disciplines represented by its staff. Is there a medical expert well-versed in chronic-pain problems and treatments? Does the clinic have properly trained therapists who can deal with the special needs of chronic-pain patients? Does the clinic offer a package of services designed to treat all the problems associated with chronic pain at the same time?

Stay away from a clinic that uses a piecemeal approach — i.e. it tries one mode of treatment at a time, hoping that eventually one will succeed. Finally, check the reputation of the clinic if you can. Do you know someone who has received help there? Have other medical experts recommended it? Have members of the clinic published serious works on chronic pain? These pointers should help you to be a smart health-care consumer.

3. *You claim to have an overall seventy per cent success rate. How do you define success? Also, why do the other thirty per cent fail?*

We judge success as follows. If a patient is able to return to work full-time, or even part-time, our treatment has succeeded. It is also successful if the patient can be retrained for another job or, if the person did not work prior to having the problem, he or she is able to resume a normal lifestyle.

Some people fail because their pain conditions just do not respond to cognitive-behavioral therapy. We have found that migraine sufferers, for example, do not respond as well as other pain sufferers.

Others may lack the commitment to follow through with the program, which requires hard work and patience. For example, they may follow the exercise programs for a while, but they neglect to modify their sleeping patterns, and they continue to take medication as needed rather than on a fixed time schedule. They simply do not understand its comprehensive nature.

4. I'm still not too sure I understand how and when acute pain becomes chronic. Is chronic pain always defined as occurring six months after the initial event?

As I mentioned in Chapter 4, nobody knows for sure why chronic pain develops. There is rarely a clear dividing line between the acute and chronic phases. The reason most experts consider chronic pain to begin six months after the onset of pain is because that is well beyond the usual healing time for an injury or illness. But it should be noted that there are other definitions, ranging from three months from the onset to six months after the *normal healing time* for an illness or injury.

But what is the usual healing time? This is a difficult question to answer, because not all parts of the body heal at the same rate. For example, injuries to the Achilles tendon take a long time to heal properly, because blood supply to that area of the leg and foot is less plentiful than elsewhere in the body. Reduced blood flow means that medications and the body's natural regeneration processes take longer to work. In general, though, it is safe to say that soft-tissue injuries heal within three months.

5. *Is chronic pain always constant, or are there periods when a person is completely pain-free?*

Many chronic-pain sufferers have continuous pain, although the intensity may vary. Others suffer from periodic bouts of pain, yet remain pain-free between episodes. Migraines or tension headaches and episodic back or neck pains fall into the latter category.

6. *My husband has a chronic-pain problem, but refuses to seek help. Nothing I say or do seems to matter. Our relationship is deteriorating. I love my spouse, but I cannot continue this way. What can I do to convince him to seek help?*

You have two problems to deal with — chronic pain, and lack of communication within your relationship. If your spouse is unwilling to listen to you and seek help for his pain problem, you must tackle your marital problems first. It is obvious that the two of you are on different wavelengths, and that you would probably benefit from marital counselling. Once the two of you overcome the difficulties in your relationship, your husband will be better able to deal with the chronic-pain condition.

7. *If the pain system can be reprogrammed using your methods, what about other "systems" in the body? What about the claims that similar therapies can cure diseases like arthritis and cancer?*

I am reluctant to propose that cognitive-behavioral therapy can help "disease" processes, although there are initial studies indicating that it may affect the body's immune systems as well as the disease process underlying rheumatoid arthritis. But we are not referring in this book to "diseases". Chronic pain seems to result from changes in *neurological function-*

ing, which *can* be affected by cognitive-behavioral therapy. We are still many years away from being able to establish one way or the other the efficacy of treating "diseases" with cognitive-behavioral therapy.

8. *You don't seem to use the term "chronic-pain syndrome" very often. Is it possible to have a chronic-pain problem but not be categorized as suffering from the syndrome?*

The majority of chronic-pain conditions are not severe enough to be classified as chronic-pain syndrome. Most individuals with pain are able to function reasonably well, unlike those with the syndrome who are unable to live or work normally. However, this is not to say that the majority without the syndrome should merely carry on without any help whatsoever. There is no reason why they should not attempt to improve the quality of their lives. Besides, they too may develop the syndrome if they go untreated.

9. *Regardless of what I say or do, nobody — including my doctors — believes me when I say I am in constant pain. They have almost convinced me that I am crazy. What can I do to convince people that my pain is real? How can I get help when everybody thinks I am only looking for attention and sympathy?*

First of all, do not try to consciously exaggerate your pain behavior (see Chapter 9) when you are with others or visiting your doctor. They will probably think you are putting on an act. Secondly, be straightforward with your doctor. Tell him of your fears and your wish to come to grips with your pain problems. If he still refuses to believe you, you should seek another medical professional — one who is more aware of the intricacies of chronic pain. Of course, if you find a health-care practitioner who specializes in chronic pain, so much the better. It may take time to find the right person, but in the long run you will be glad you made the effort.

10. *Your comments about exercise make sense to me, but I am puzzled by the difficulties I am having with exercise. Why is it that my muscles often cramp up after I have been exercising?*

If you have a chronic-pain condition, and are just now beginning to exercise again, you may be abusing your muscles. Perhaps you are doing too much too soon. Have you followed your baseline, shaping, pacing program? You may have to return to your baseline and start over. Also, you may not be exercising properly and could use the help of a physiotherapist who can teach you how to warm up and cool down properly. It is very important to stretch out the muscles both before and after you do your exercises.

11. *You talk mainly about "controlling", "managing", and "coping with" chronic pain. Does this mean that some people are totally "cured" while others have to settle for a mere "improvement" in their condition?*

In a follow-up study of our patients, over twelve per cent of them reported that they were totally pain-free a year and a half after completing our treatment program. Successful patients reported a fifty six per cent reduction in pain. Others said that they still had the same amount of pain, *but* stated that they felt much better. The three primary reasons the latter patients gave for this were: (a) they were better able to cope with the pain; (b) the pain just did not bother them as much as before; and (c) they discovered that they could do more despite their discomfort. This last finding is important, because increased activity is usually associated with *increased* pain. Therefore, this finding could be considered tantamount to having *less* pain.

Yes, we wish that the percentage of pain-free patients could be higher, and perhaps it will be when we learn more about the pain system. In the meantime, the patients we classify as successes are quite pleased with the reductions in their pain levels and their increased levels of activity.

12. *I suffer from migraine headaches, which begin about the same time every year and last for five weeks. This has gone on for many years. Is there anything I can do to avoid them? If they do begin again, how can I cope with them, without taking stupefying drugs, when I know they will last for more than a month?*

There are many known causes of migraine headaches, which as you describe them, are often referred to as "cluster headaches". You can take certain steps to minimize your chances of getting them. The most common triggers seem to be significant changes in the weather, certain foods, and stress. While it may be difficult for you to do anything about the climate, you can learn more about possible food reactions, and you can certainly use cognitive-behavioral methods to monitor and control your stress and anxiety levels. There are migraine headache associations in Canada and the United States, and you may want to get in touch with one of them for more information. You should see a headache specialist if you haven't already.

13. *Is it possible for me to control my pain so well that I might forget about my physical limitations and do something to harm myself?*

Cognitive-behavioral therapy is not so powerful that you will completely forget that you once had a serious pain problem. If you have any lingering concerns about your physical condition, you should have a complete medical examination to clarify your situation. Of course, it is impossible to predict what can happen to you, but you should try not to worry about the potential of another serious accident. The fear of reinjuring yourself could lead you to adopt a more invalid-like lifestyle which can in fact increase your current pain levels.

14. *Suppose I hurt myself or develop a painful illness. Is*

*there anything I can do to avoid developing chronic-pain
syndrome?*

The simple answer is "yes". Now that you are familiar with
the symptoms associated with chronic-pain syndrome, and
how to deal with those symptoms, you should be able to
identify and prevent them from developing. If you feel that
you are falling into a chronic-pain trap, monitor yourself
carefully. Is your behavior changing? Are you adopting a
more sedentary lifestyle? Are you having trouble falling
asleep? Are you taking a lot of painkilling medication?

If the answer to these questions is affirmative, you can
begin to practice the techniques outlined in this book. If you
attack the problem before it becomes entrenched, you should
succeed in avoiding the problem. It is far easier to prevent
chronic-pain syndrome than to cure it.

Glossary

Active Therapies: Therapies in which the patient is an active collaborator and participant in the therapeutic process (cf. Passive Therapies).

Acupuncture: An ancient Chinese technique for the stimulation of peripheral nerves either with needles or, more recently, with a low-power laser.

Acute Pain: Short-term severe pain which rarely lasts more than a few hours, or at most a few days.

Adequate Therapeutic Trial: The principle that each therapy should have an optimal time frame to determine its effectiveness.

Analgesics: Medications which have the primary effect of reducing pain.

Anti-Inflammatory Medication: Medication which has the major effect of reducing inflammation (e.g. Feldene, Orudis). Most anti-inflammatories also have an analgesic effect.

Anxiolytic: An activity or medication which reduces anxiety.

Assertiveness: A direct way of stating one's needs, wants, and desires to produce changes in one's environment. Not to be confused with aggressiveness.

Audio Focusing: Concentrating on verbal or other auditory stimulation as a relaxation technique.

Autogenic Relaxation: A relaxation technique that focuses on the various sensations that are experienced during the process of relaxation, e.g. warmth, lightness.

Axon: The part of a nerve cell along which the electrical impulse travels.

Baseline: As used in this book, a measure of the amount of an activity that produces a noticeable increase in pain.

Biofeedback: A technique of measuring physiological responses that are not usually consciously available to a person. The information is then fed back to the individual in a form that allows him or her to learn how to modify the physiological response.

Central Nervous System: The sum total of nerve tissue within the spinal cord and the brain.

Chronic Pain: Pain usually defined as persisting for at least six months.

Chronic-Pain Syndrome: A constellation of behavioral, emotional, physical, and cognitive changes that accompany chronic pain and serve to worsen the pain and the disability.

Cognition: The process of thinking and knowing, including perception, memory, judgement, and so on. This includes thoughts, ideas, beliefs, and attitudes.

Cognitive-Behavioral Therapy: A systematic learning approach to a range of human problems focusing here on pain therapy. Cognitive-behavioral therapy is derived from learning principles in psychology.

Cognitive Dissonance: A state of inner turmoil resulting from contradictions in a person's beliefs or contradictions between beliefs and behavior.

Cognitive Restructuring: A systematic process of uncovering and modifying cognitions. Used in cognitive-behavioral therapy.

Conditioned Responses: Behaviors produced because of past learning, either through operant or classical conditioning.

Dependence: The unhealthy need for a medication or a treatment.

Disease Model: An approach utilized by the medical profession in which complaints or "symptoms" are seen as rooted in disease or injury.

Distraction: An imagery technique in which one's attention is focused away from the undesirable stimulus.

Dorsal Horn: A part of the spinal cord where there are numerous nerve connections that are proposed to make up the "gate mechanism".

Endorphins: Morphine-like substances which exist in our brains and bodies.

Focusing: An imagery technique in which one's attention is concentrated on modifying the undesirable sensation.

Imagery: Models of the real world created in your mind using any of the senses. These can occur spontaneously or can be consciously produced.

Learned Helplessness: A state akin to depression, in which inactive, lethargic behavior interferes with normal learning.

Learned Pain: Pain produced by the central nervous system because of past reinforcements and conditioning. Also known as "memorized pain".

Local Anesthetic: A pain-killing chemical which is usually injected to deaden pain in a particular area, e.g. the use of Novocain by dentists.

Malingering: The conscious exaggeration or "faking" of a pain state or other symptoms.

Motor Signals: Messages sent from the central nervous system to peripheral muscles that produce muscular activity.

Multi-Dimensional Treatment: A perspective and therapeutic approach which encompasses all of the contributing elements of a problem.

Neurochemicals: Specialized chemicals which exist in and around the synapse and convey messages from one nerve cell to the other.

Operant Pain: Pain produced through reinforcement of pain behaviors.

Pacing: The process of controlling activities based upon predetermined schedules, as opposed to having those activities controlled by pain levels.

Pain-Control Strategy: Any technique or approach used by a person to manage pain.

Pain Cue: A feeling of tightness or mild discomfort which predictably signals the onset of a pain increase and which can be used as a cue for pacing.

Pain-Prone Personality: A theoretical construct that some people are prone to developing pain conditions.

Pain Scale: A way of reporting the amount of pain experienced such as the 0 to 10 scale used in this book.

Pain System: The nervous-system pathways that serve to signal damage and create the perception of pain.

Pain Threshold: This indicates the level at which pain begins to intrude into conscious awareness. Pain may be in existence below the threshold level, but the individual may not be constantly aware of it.

Pain Tolerance: The point at which pain becomes so severe that it significantly interferes with activities.

Pain-Triggers: Factors such as emotions, stress, physical activity, etc. that serve to modify the functioning of the pain system and thereby the experience of pain.

Passive Therapies: Treatment techniques in which the patients is a passive recipient of care, e.g. massage, TENS, etc.

Phantom-Limb Pain: Pain in a limb or extremity that has been amputated.

Phobia: An unreasonable fear of a thing, situation, or other stimulus.

Placebo: A "fake" treatment such as a sugar pill which is given to a patient who believes that the treatment is in fact real.

Post-Traumatic Stress Disorder: A diagnosis for a person experiencing the emotional sequelae of a traumatic event such as an accident or a wartime experience. It is characterized by frequent rumination on the traumatic event, nightmares, and anxiety attacks. Pain may also be a symptom.

Psoriatic Arthritis: One of more than a hundred arthritic conditions. It is associated with psoriasis.

Re-Labelling: An imagery technique in which one focuses on directly modifying the perception and experience of a negative stimulus.

Self-Hypnosis: Hypnosis which is conducted and controlled by the individual.

Self-Talk: The inner voice that helps us to monitor our actions and direct our activities.

Shaping: The process of taking small, predetermined, and graduated steps to increase the amount of an activity.

Sleep-Onset Insomnia: A persistent inability to fall asleep at the desired bedtime.

Soft-Tissue Injury: An injury to muscle, tendons, or ligaments, as distinct from an injury to bones or nerves.

Spontaneous Remission: An automatic recovery process that occurs with any injury or disease.

Synapse: The point at which two nerve cells communicate with each other through the release and uptake of neurochemicals.

Systematic Desensitization: Consists of pairing a relaxed state with the imagined or real presentation of the phobic stimulus with the result that the stimulus gradually fails to elicit the fear response.

Thought-Stopping: Using a sharp, predetermined command to yourself to stop undesirable thoughts or activities. The command can either be under your breath or spoken out loud.

Transcutaneous Electrical Nerve Stimulation (TENS):   An electrical stimulator placed upon various points on the skin which has the effect of temporarily reducing pain.

Type-A Personality: A theoretical construct of a personality type who is aggressive, highly stressed, success- and achievement-oriented, uptight, anxious, and obsessive about details. There are indications that Type-A persons may be more susceptible to cardiovascular disease and stress-related illnesses.

Working to Schedule: Pacing an activity according to a predetermined limit, independent of pain.

Working to Tolerance: Engaging in an activity and pushing to your level of conditioning, i.e. your physical stamina or pain level.

Suggested Reading

1. Benson, Herbert, M.D., *The Relaxation Response*. New York: Avon Books, 1976.
2. Bergland, Richard, M.D., *The Fabric of Mind*. New York: Viking Penguin, 1986.
3. Bresler, David E., M.D. (with Richard Trubo), *Free Yourself from Pain*. New York: Simon & Schuster, 1979.
4. Cousins, Norman, *Anatomy of an Illness*. New York: Bantam Books, 1981.
5. Hall, Hamilton, M.D., *More Advice from the Back Doctor*. Toronto: McClelland and Stewart, 1987.
6. Melzack, Ronald, and Patrick Wall, *The Challenge of Pain*. Toronto: Penguin Books, 1984.
7. Turk, D. C., D. Meikenbaum, and M. Genest, *Pain and Behavioral Medicine: A Cognitive-Behavioral Perspective*. New York: Guilford Press, 1983.

Index

There's an epidemic with 27 million victims. And no visible symptoms.

It's an epidemic of people who can't read.

Believe it or not, 27 million Americans are functionally illiterate, about one adult in five.

The solution to this problem is you... when you join the fight against illiteracy. So call the Coalition for Literacy at toll-free **1-800-228-8813** and volunteer.

Volunteer Against Illiteracy. The only degree you need is a degree of caring.